My Cancer Journey

Kicking

Cancer's

Butt!!

Dianne Terry

Réalta Publications

Published by Réalta Publications in 2019

First Edition; First printing

Design and writing by Dianne Terry

ISBN: 978-0-9600417-6-3

This Journal belongs to

_____

If found, please call

_____

In Case of Emergency, please call

_____

_____

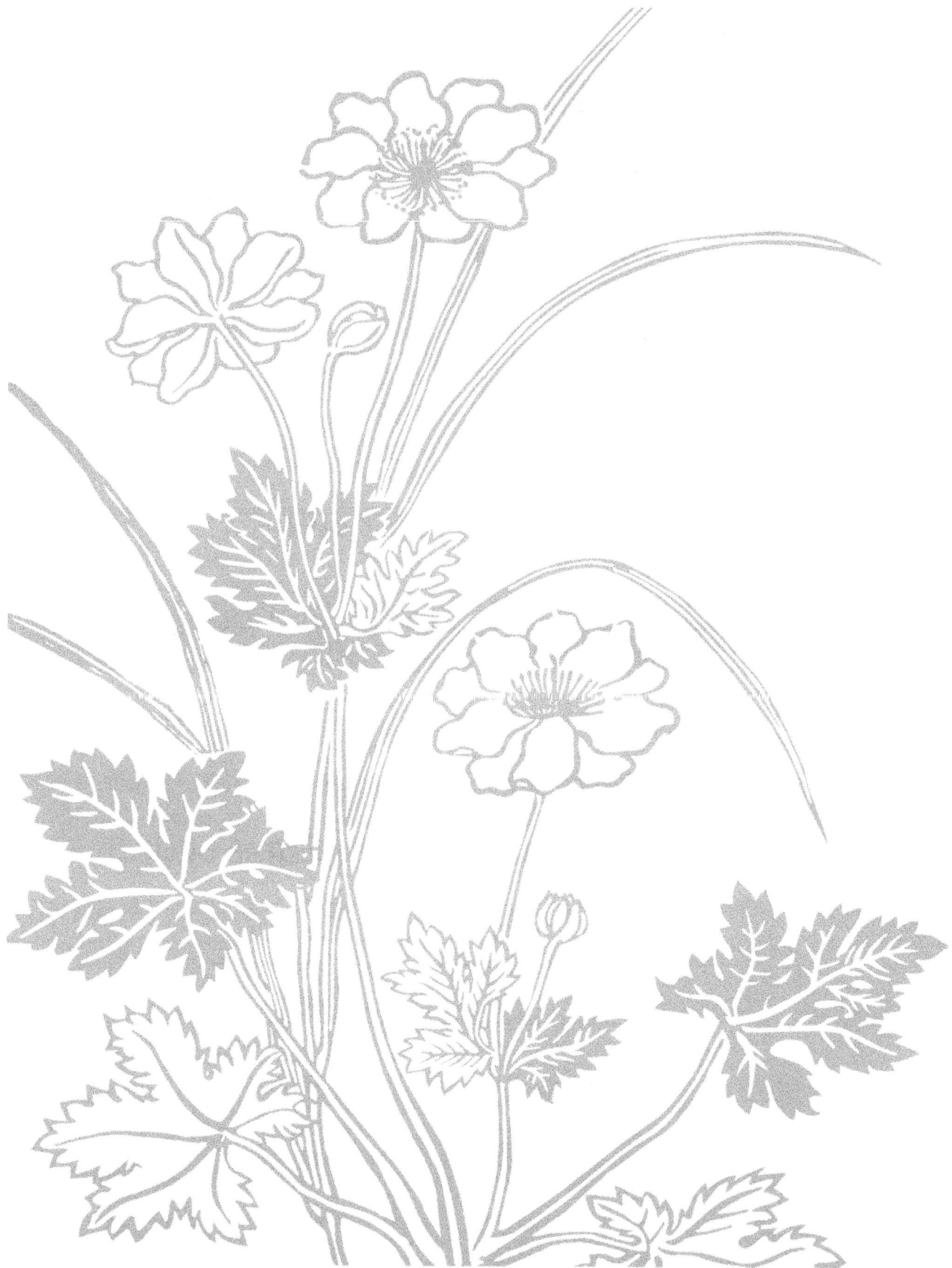

Dedication

This book is dedicated to all the
people who have and will endure
the seemingly endless treatments
for the insidious disease called

CANCER.

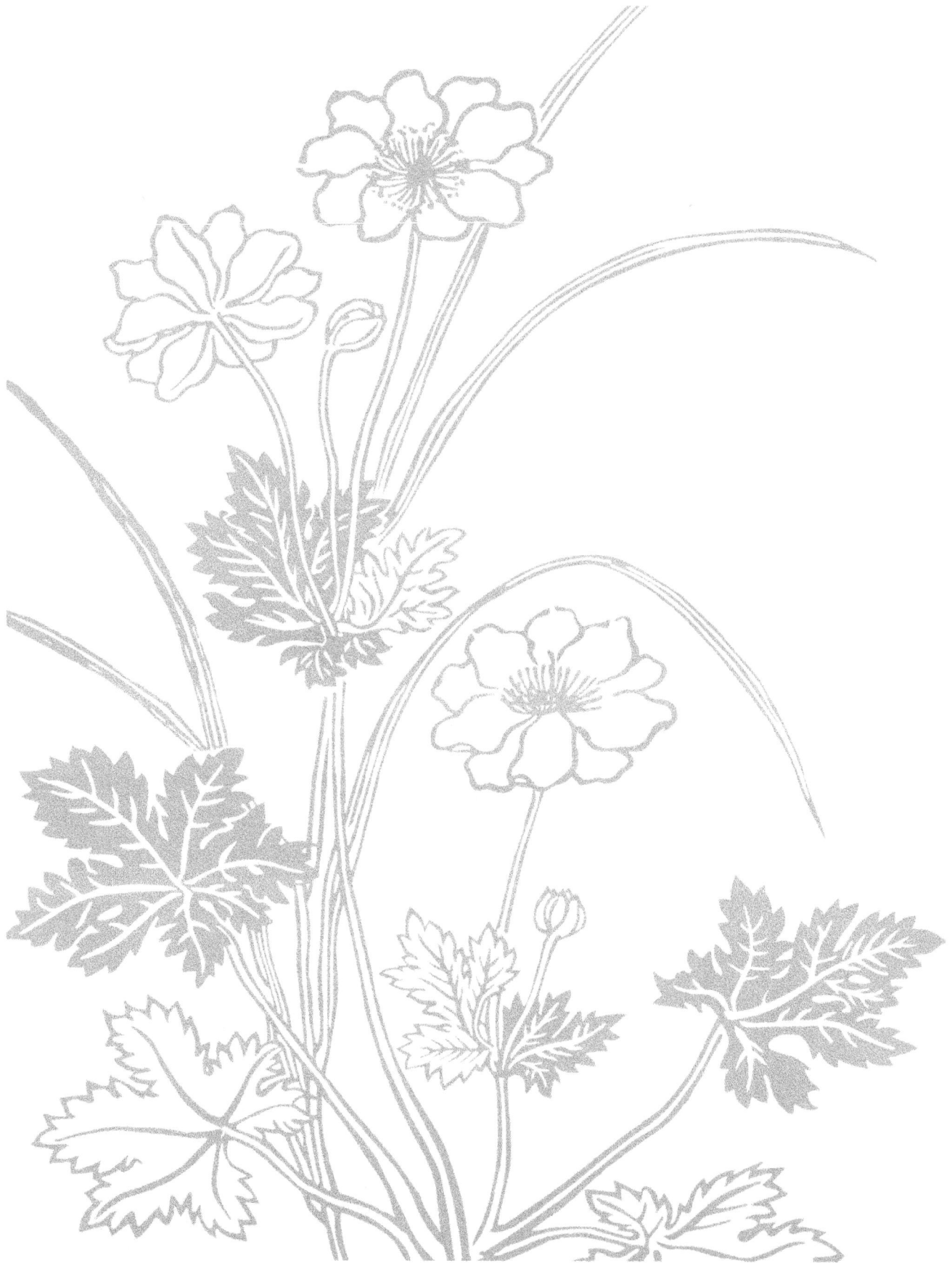

Table of Contents

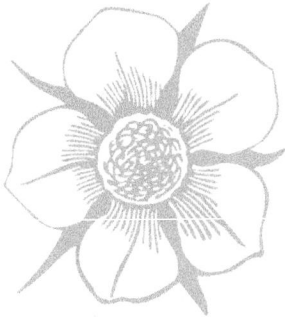

A Personal Note to You

Hearing the words "You have CANCER" is probably one of the scariest, most devastating things you will ever experience. It feels like your heart actually stops beating in your chest for a moment. You may feel like crying or even screaming.

Thoughts of all the things you wanted to do but may not have time for now . . . You've been dreading hearing that word ever since you started down this road, even though you kept pushing it down—never saying "that word" out loud.

I can't take away your cancer, but I hope this journal will provide some resources and assurances for you. It is designed to help you capture important information about **you**: your health, your doctors, your visits for treatments, and especially how you **feel** during this journey from diagnosis to **cure**.

My sincere prayer and hope for you is this journal provides the "one-stop-shopping" you need as you embark on this journey. I'm not talking about the purchase of this journal—I'm talking about being able to corral everything you need to remember into one spot so you only have to pick up your journal as you get ready to head out the door to the next round of chemo or consultations.

One of the things we've noticed after dealing with cancer is "chemo brain" which seems to affect many if not all cancer patients. It's a fuzzy phenomenon that keeps you from being able to make sense of the simplest tasks. Perhaps it's just overwhelm, but more likely "chemo brain" is caused by the very treatment you are receiving. Because of this, it's hard to focus, be organized . . . and think of anything past survival.

It's hard to remember what you need to ask the doctor, what he tells you, special instructions about medications—so many things.

Whatever the cause for "chemo brain", simplifying your life is key to getting through all this and remaining sane. :)

Now, just so we're clear here—I'm not promising sanity, but if you keep things together —*as best you can*—and stay **positive**, you may find you are able to handle the ups and downs better.

> When you're dealing with cancer, a daily dose of inspiration may make a big difference in your outlook on life.

Keeping a positive outlook is proven to help with stress management, but when someone says to "think positive" or "be optimistic" during a time such as cancer, it can be much easier said than done.

I know cancer isn't all rainbow and butterflies and once you enter a dark mindset, it can be hard to get out of it. But most of us have that *one message* of hope and inspiration that somehow manages to help bring some perspective and optimism to the situation.

No one "deserves" cancer, and least of all you. So let's get started on this journey. On the next page, you will find instructions for how to get the best use of this journal.

How to Use This Journal

1. Commit to fighting this disease. Don't let it define you. FIGHT.

2. Don't fight alone. Enlist the help and support of your friends and family. They would be willing to take you to treatments when you don't feel like driving. They will pray with and for you. Take all the help you can get. Build your village with people who care about you.

3. Fill out the important information at the front of this journal as soon as you can. You will be using some of it at every appointment.

4. We all have a different path that leads us to the cancer diagnosis. Your story is important. Write about your journey to diagnosis. It may save the life of someone in your family some day—when they read about your first symptoms.

5. Important medical information is just that—fill out your blood type, medical alert, allergies and any surgeries you've had.

6. There are two pages for medical insurance—maybe too many for you, but fill in all applicable. Don't forget dental, eyeglasses, cancer insurance and anything else that comes to mind.

7. Medications—both prescriptions and over-the-counter vitamins and supplements. Your medical team will need all of this information to determine if anything you take affects or is affected by your prescribed treatments (chemo, etc.)

8. Write down all your doctors. It is important to have contact information for each of them so they can all be aware of your treatments. And yes, it is important for even your optometrist and dentist to be aware of what is going on with your health.

9. **Always** take this journal with you to doctor appointments or when going for treatments. By taking this along and keeping it up-to-date, you will have a record of all your questions, doctor instructions, blood tests . . . IN ONE PLACE.

How to Use This Journal (cont'd)

10. Capture your questions during the week to ask the doctor on your next visit. Then write down his responses and instructions.

11. Take time to write down how you feel each day—physically and emotionally.

12. Keep track of any side-effects you have to medications prescribed to you. Report those to the doctor when you see him next.

13. There's a year's worth of monthly calendar so you can keep track of important dates and events.

14. Two pages are provided for each doctor / treatment visit.

15. Twenty-six weeks of journaling is provided—one page for each week. Write about how you felt that day.

16. Twenty-six pages that include an inspirational saying and a picture are provided for encouragement. Take your coloring pencils along with you when you go for your appointments. It's the perfect way to relieve stress as you wait for an appointment or while receiving treatments.

17. Last . . . **but most important** . . . Be sure to focus on positives. Remember, even though chemo is running through your body, it is finding and attacking cancer cells—killing each one so it can no longer affect you.

This is how my journey began

I first noticed:

My first doctor's appointment:

The journey to diagnosis:

Diagnosis

My diagnosis was made on _____

When I heard the news, I felt _____

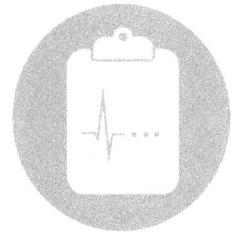

_____

_____

_____

MY F.I.G.H.T. Plan

I realize that it's MY responsibility to fight this cancer growing inside me. Here are some things I will do to ensure victory:

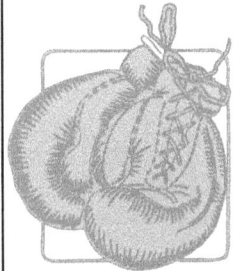

I. AM.

CANCER.FREE!!!!

Today's Date _____

Cancer is a <u>WORD</u>,
not a sentence.

—John Diamond

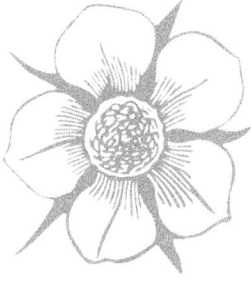

Important Medical Information

My Blood Type: _____

Medical Alert Information: _____
_____
_____
_____
_____

I am allergic to: _____
_____
_____
_____

Previous Surgeries:

Date: _____ Surgeon: _____
Surgery: _____
_____

Date: _____ Surgeon: _____
Surgery: _____
_____

Date: _____ Surgeon: _____
Surgery: _____
_____

Date: _____ Surgeon: _____
Surgery: _____
_____

Date: _____ Surgeon: _____
Surgery: _____
_____

My Medical History

	Rheumatic Fever		Lung (Pulmonary Disease)
	Heart Disease		COPD
	Heart Attack >50		Water on the Lungs
	Heart Attack <50		Asthma
	High Blood Pressure		Type I Diabetes
	AFib—Atrial Fibrillation		Type II Diabetes
	Pacemaker		Type III Diabetes
	Heart Murmur		Hepatitis A, B, or C
	High Cholesterol		Headaches/Migraines (w/aura)
	Stroke		Headaches/Migraines (w/out aura)
	Whooping Cough (Pertussis)		Seizure Disorder
	Measles		Epilepsy
	Meningitis		Digestive Tract
	Chicken Pox (Varicella)		Gallbladder/Gallstones
	Mumps		Diabetes
	Pneumonia		Liver Disease / Hepatitis
	Polio		Thyroid
	Tuberculosis		Kidney Renal Disease
	HIV Infection		Kidney Stones
	Eczema		Prostate Problems
	Tattoo		Rheumatoid Arthritis
	Hay Fever		Prior Orthopedic Problems
	Hives (Uticaria)		Joint Problems
	Allergies		Depression / Suicide
	Ear/Nose/Throat		Alcoholism
	Hearing Problems		Drug Addiction
	Immune Disorder		Anxiety

My Medical History (cont'd)

	Skin Cancer		Panic Attacks
	Cancer		Mental Health Disorder
	Anemia		Fertility
	Hernia: Type _____		Colon Polyps? _____
			Type: _____

My Family Medical History

Condition	* G/A/U C/P/S	Condition	* G/A/U C/P/S
Heart Disease		Cancer	
Heart Attack		Breast	
High Blood Pressure		Colorectal	
High Cholesterol		Lung	
Kidney Disease		Prostate / Ovarian	
Lung Disease		Skin	
Asthma		Other: _____	
COPD		Liver Disease	
Migraines		Stroke	
Dementia		Tuberculosis	
Alzheimers		Depression/Suicide	
Mental Disorder		Epilepsy/Seizures	
Thyroid Disease		Diabetes	
Smokers		Alcoholism	
Osteoporosis		Drug Addiction	

Doctors and Hospitals

HOSPITAL: _____
Address:_____
_____
City/State/Zip:_____
Phone:_____ Fax:_____

PRIMARY CARE: _____
Address: _____
_____
City/State/Zip: _____
Phone: _____ Fax: _____

OB-GYN: _____
Address: _____
_____
City/State/Zip:_____
Phone:_____ Fax: _____

DENTIST: _____
Address: _____
_____
City/State/Zip: _____
Phone: _____ Fax: _____

OPTOMETRIST: _____
Address:_____
_____
City/State/Zip: _____
Phone: _____ Fax: _____

SPECIALIST: _____
Address:_____
_____
City/State/Zip:_____
Phone: _____ Fax: _____

Doctors and Hospitals

SPECIALIST: _____
Address:_____
_____
City/State/Zip:_____
Phone: _____ Fax: _____

SPECIALIST: _____
Address:_____
_____
City/State/Zip:_____
Phone: _____ Fax: _____

SPECIALIST: _____
Address:_____
_____
City/State/Zip:_____
Phone: _____ Fax: _____

SPECIALIST: _____
Address:_____
_____
City/State/Zip:_____
Phone: _____ Fax: _____

SPECIALIST: _____
Address:_____
_____
City/State/Zip:_____
Phone: _____ Fax: _____

SPECIALIST: _____
Address:_____
_____
City/State/Zip:_____
Phone: _____ Fax: _____

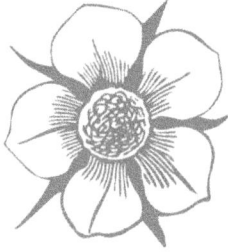

Medical Insurance

Primary Insurance: _____

Policy #: _____

Policy Start Date:_____ **Policy End Date:**_____

Address: _____

City/State/Zip: _____

Contact: _____

Phone: _____

Email:_____

Secondary Insurance: _____

Policy #: _____

Policy Start Date:_____ **Policy End Date:**_____

Address: _____

City/State/Zip: _____

Contact: _____

Phone: _____

Email:_____

Additional Insurance: _____

Policy #: _____

Policy Start Date:_____ **Policy End Date:**_____

Address: _____

City/State/Zip: _____

Contact: _____

Phone: _____

Email:_____

Additional Insurance: _____

Policy #: _____

Policy Start Date:_____ **Policy End Date:**_____

Address: _____

City/State/Zip: _____

Contact: _____

Phone: _____

Email:_____

Additional Medical Insurance

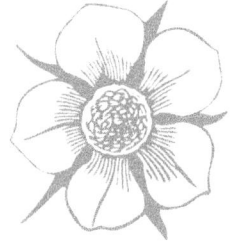

Additional Insurance: _____

Policy #: _____

Policy Start Date:_____ Policy End Date:_____

Address: _____

City/State/Zip: _____

Contact: _____

Phone: _____

Email:_____

Additional Insurance: _____

Policy #: _____

Policy Start Date:_____ Policy End Date:_____

Address: _____

City/State/Zip: _____

Contact: _____

Phone: _____

Email:_____

Additional Insurance: _____

Policy #: _____

Policy Start Date:_____ Policy End Date:_____

Address: _____

City/State/Zip: _____

Contact: _____

Phone: _____

Email:_____

Additional Insurance: _____

Policy #: _____

Policy Start Date:_____ Policy End Date:_____

Address: _____

City/State/Zip: _____

Contact: _____

Phone: _____

Email:_____

My Medications

Prescriptions

Name	Dosage	Frequency	What's it For?

My Medications

Vitamins and Supplements

Name	Dosage	Frequency	What's it For?

Calendar

Year: _____

Monday	Tuesday	Wednesday
☐	☐	☐
☐	☐	☐
☐	☐	☐
☐	☐	☐
☐	☐	☐

Notes: _____
_____
_____
_____
_____
_____
_____
_____

Calendar

Month: _____

Thursday	Friday	Saturday
		Sunday
☐	☐	☐
		☐
☐	☐	☐
		☐
☐	☐	☐
		☐
☐	☐	☐
		☐
☐	☐	☐
		☐

Notes: _____
_____
_____
_____
_____
_____
_____
_____

Calendar

Year: _____

Monday	Tuesday	Wednesday
☐	☐	☐
☐	☐	☐
☐	☐	☐
☐	☐	☐
☐	☐	☐

Notes: _____
_____
_____
_____
_____
_____
_____
_____
_____

Calendar

Month: _____

Thursday	Friday	Saturday
		Sunday
☐	☐	☐ ☐
☐	☐	☐ ☐
☐	☐	☐ ☐
☐	☐	☐ ☐
☐	☐	☐ ☐

Notes: _____
_____
_____
_____
_____
_____
_____
_____

Calendar

Year: _____

Monday	Tuesday	Wednesday
☐	☐	☐
☐	☐	☐
☐	☐	☐
☐	☐	☐
☐	☐	☐

Notes: _____
_____
_____
_____
_____
_____
_____
_____

Calendar

Month: _____

Thursday	Friday	Saturday
		Sunday
☐	☐	☐ ☐
☐	☐	☐ ☐
☐	☐	☐ ☐
☐	☐	☐ ☐
☐	☐	☐ ☐

Notes: _____

_____

_____

_____

_____

_____

_____

Calendar

Year: _____

Monday	Tuesday	Wednesday
☐	☐	☐
☐	☐	☐
☐	☐	☐
☐	☐	☐
☐	☐	☐

Notes: _____
_____
_____
_____
_____
_____
_____
_____

Calendar

Month: _____

Thursday	Friday	Saturday
		Sunday
☐	☐	☐
		☐
☐	☐	☐
		☐
☐	☐	☐
		☐
☐	☐	☐
		☐
☐	☐	☐
		☐

Notes: _____
_____
_____
_____
_____
_____
_____
_____

Calendar

Year: _____

Monday	Tuesday	Wednesday
☐	☐	☐
☐	☐	☐
☐	☐	☐
☐	☐	☐
☐	☐	☐

Notes: _____

_____

_____

_____

_____

_____

_____

_____

Calendar

Month: _____

Thursday	Friday	Saturday
		Sunday
☐	☐	☐ ☐
☐	☐	☐ ☐
☐	☐	☐ ☐
☐	☐	☐ ☐
☐	☐	☐ ☐

Notes: _____
_____
_____
_____
_____
_____
_____
_____

Calendar

Year: _____

Monday	Tuesday	Wednesday
☐	☐	☐
☐	☐	☐
☐	☐	☐
☐	☐	☐
☐	☐	☐

Notes: _____
_____
_____
_____
_____
_____
_____
_____

Calendar

Month: _____

Thursday	Friday	Saturday
		Sunday
☐	☐	☐ _____ ☐
☐	☐	☐ _____ ☐
☐	☐	☐ _____ ☐
☐	☐	☐ _____ ☐
☐	☐	☐ _____ ☐

Notes: _____
_____
_____
_____
_____
_____
_____
_____

Calendar

Year: _____

Monday	Tuesday	Wednesday
☐	☐	☐
☐	☐	☐
☐	☐	☐
☐	☐	☐
☐	☐	☐

Notes: _____
_____
_____
_____
_____
_____
_____
_____

Calendar

Month: _____

Thursday	Friday	Saturday
		Sunday
☐	☐	☐
		☐
☐	☐	☐
		☐
☐	☐	☐
		☐
☐	☐	☐
		☐
☐	☐	☐
		☐

Notes: _____
_____
_____
_____
_____
_____
_____
_____

Calendar

Year: _____

Monday	Tuesday	Wednesday
☐	☐	☐
☐	☐	☐
☐	☐	☐
☐	☐	☐
☐	☐	☐

Notes: _____
_____
_____
_____
_____
_____
_____
_____

Calendar

Month: _____

Thursday	Friday	Saturday
		Sunday
☐	☐	☐
		☐
☐	☐	☐
		☐
☐	☐	☐
		☐
☐	☐	☐
		☐
☐	☐	☐
		☐

Notes: _____
_____
_____
_____
_____
_____
_____
_____

Calendar

Year: _____

Monday	Tuesday	Wednesday
☐	☐	☐
☐	☐	☐
☐	☐	☐
☐	☐	☐
☐	☐	☐

Notes: _____
_____
_____
_____
_____
_____
_____
_____

Calendar

Month: _____

Thursday	Friday	Saturday
		Sunday
☐	☐	☐
		☐
☐	☐	☐
		☐
☐	☐	☐
		☐
☐	☐	☐
		☐
☐	☐	☐
		☐

Notes: _____
_____
_____
_____
_____
_____
_____
_____

Calendar

Year: _____

Monday	Tuesday	Wednesday
☐	☐	☐
☐	☐	☐
☐	☐	☐
☐	☐	☐
☐	☐	☐

Notes: _____
_____
_____
_____
_____
_____
_____
_____

Calendar

Month: _____

Thursday	Friday	Saturday / Sunday
☐	☐	☐ ☐
☐	☐	☐ ☐
☐	☐	☐ ☐
☐	☐	☐ ☐
☐	☐	☐ ☐

Notes: _____
_____
_____
_____
_____
_____
_____
_____

Calendar

Year: _____

Monday	Tuesday	Wednesday
☐	☐	☐
☐	☐	☐
☐	☐	☐
☐	☐	☐
☐	☐	☐

Notes: _____
_____
_____
_____
_____
_____
_____
_____

Calendar

Month: _____

Thursday	Friday	Saturday
		Sunday
☐	☐	☐
		☐
☐	☐	☐
		☐
☐	☐	☐
		☐
☐	☐	☐
		☐
☐	☐	☐
		☐

Notes: _____
_____
_____
_____
_____
_____
_____
_____

Calendar

Year: _____

Monday	Tuesday	Wednesday
☐	☐	☐
☐	☐	☐
☐	☐	☐
☐	☐	☐
☐	☐	☐

Notes: _____

_____

_____

_____

_____

_____

_____

_____

Calendar

Month: _____

Thursday	Friday	Saturday
		Sunday
☐	☐	☐ ☐
☐	☐	☐ ☐
☐	☐	☐ ☐
☐	☐	☐ ☐
☐	☐	☐ ☐

Notes: _____
_____
_____
_____
_____
_____
_____
_____

Office Visit

Date/Time: _____

Doctor: _____

Reason for Visit: _____

Blood Cell Count

White Blood Cell	Red Blood Cell
Hemoglobin	Hematocrit
Platelets	Other

Questions to ask the doctor: _____

_____

_____

_____

_____

_____

_____

Doctor's Diagnosis/Feedback: _____

_____

_____

_____

_____

Treatment Received Today: _____

_____

_____

Any medication changes? _____

_____

_____

Office Visit

Next Visit

Date/Time _____

Purpose _____

Who will I see? _____

Today I'm feeling:

    O   Better   O   Worse   O   Same

    O   Pain   O   Fatigue   O   Depression

NOTES

Office Visit

Date/Time: _____

Doctor: _____

Reason for Visit: _____

Blood Cell Count

White Blood Cell	Red Blood Cell
Hemoglobin	Hematocrit
Platelets	Other

Questions to ask the doctor: _____
_____
_____
_____
_____
_____
_____

Doctor's Diagnosis/Feedback: _____
_____
_____
_____

Treatment Received Today: _____
_____
_____

Any medication changes? _____
_____
_____

Next Visit

Date/Time _____

Purpose _____

Who will I see? _____

Today I'm feeling:

O Better   O Worse   O Same

O Pain   O Fatigue   O Depression

NOTES

Office Visit

Date/Time: _____

Doctor: _____

Reason for Visit: _____

Blood Cell Count

White Blood Cell	Red Blood Cell
Hemoglobin	Hematocrit
Platelets	Other

Questions to ask the doctor: _____
_____
_____
_____
_____
_____
_____

Doctor's Diagnosis/Feedback: _____
_____
_____
_____
_____

Treatment Received Today: _____
_____
_____

Any medication changes? _____
_____
_____

Next Visit

Date/Time _____

Purpose _____

Who will I see? _____

Today I'm feeling:

- ◯ Better
- ◯ Worse
- ◯ Same
- ◯ Pain
- ◯ Fatigue
- ◯ Depression

NOTES

Office Visit

Date/Time: _____

Doctor: _____

Reason for Visit: _____

Blood Cell Count

White Blood Cell	Red Blood Cell
Hemoglobin	Hematocrit
Platelets	Other

Questions to ask the doctor: _____
_____
_____
_____
_____
_____
_____

Doctor's Diagnosis/Feedback: _____
_____
_____
_____
_____

Treatment Received Today: _____
_____
_____

Any medication changes? _____
_____
_____

Next Visit

Date/Time _____

Purpose _____

Who will I see? _____

Today I'm feeling:

O Better   O Worse   O Same

O Pain   O Fatigue   O Depression

NOTES

Office Visit	Date/Time: _____
	Doctor: _____

Reason for Visit: _____

Blood Cell Count

White Blood Cell	Red Blood Cell
Hemoglobin	Hematocrit
Platelets	Other

Questions to ask the doctor: _____
_____
_____
_____
_____
_____
_____

Doctor's Diagnosis/Feedback: _____
_____
_____
_____
_____

Treatment Received Today: _____
_____
_____

Any medication changes? _____
_____
_____

Office Visit

Next Visit

Date/Time _____

Purpose _____

Who will I see? _____

Today I'm feeling:

- O Better
- O Worse
- O Same
- O Pain
- O Fatigue
- O Depression

NOTES

Office Visit

Date/Time: _____

Doctor: _____

Reason for Visit: _____

Blood Cell Count

White Blood Cell	Red Blood Cell
Hemoglobin	Hematocrit
Platelets	Other

Questions to ask the doctor: _____
_____
_____
_____
_____
_____
_____

Doctor's Diagnosis/Feedback: _____
_____
_____
_____
_____

Treatment Received Today: _____
_____
_____

Any medication changes? _____
_____
_____

Next Visit

Date/Time _____

Purpose _____

Who will I see? _____

Today I'm feeling:

O   Better   O   Worse   O   Same

O   Pain   O   Fatigue   O   Depression

NOTES

Office Visit

Date/Time: _____

Doctor: _____

Reason for Visit: _____

Blood Cell Count

White Blood Cell	Red Blood Cell
Hemoglobin	Hematocrit
Platelets	Other

Questions to ask the doctor: _____
_____
_____
_____
_____
_____
_____

Doctor's Diagnosis/Feedback: _____
_____
_____
_____
_____

Treatment Received Today: _____
_____
_____

Any medication changes? _____
_____
_____

Next Visit

Date/Time _____

Purpose _____

Who will I see? _____

Today I'm feeling:

O   Better   O   Worse   O   Same

O   Pain   O   Fatigue   O   Depression

NOTES

Office Visit

Date/Time: _____

Doctor: _____

Reason for Visit: _____

Blood Cell Count

White Blood Cell	Red Blood Cell
Hemoglobin	Hematocrit
Platelets	Other

Questions to ask the doctor: _____

_____

_____

_____

_____

_____

_____

Doctor's Diagnosis/Feedback: _____

_____

_____

_____

Treatment Received Today: _____

_____

_____

Any medication changes? _____

_____

_____

Next Visit

Date/Time _____

Purpose _____

Who will I see? _____

Today I'm feeling:

○ Better   ○ Worse   ○ Same

○ Pain   ○ Fatigue   ○ Depression

NOTES

Office Visit

Date/Time: _____

Doctor: _____

Reason for Visit: _____

Blood Cell Count

White Blood Cell	Red Blood Cell
Hemoglobin	Hematocrit
Platelets	Other

Questions to ask the doctor: _____

_____

_____

_____

_____

_____

_____

Doctor's Diagnosis/Feedback: _____

_____

_____

_____

_____

Treatment Received Today: _____

_____

_____

Any medication changes? _____

_____

_____

Office Visit

Next Visit

Date/Time _____

Purpose _____

Who will I see? _____

Today I'm feeling:

- ◯ Better
- ◯ Pain
- ◯ Worse
- ◯ Fatigue
- ◯ Same
- ◯ Depression

NOTES

Office Visit

Date/Time: _____

Doctor: _____

Reason for Visit: _____

Blood Cell Count

White Blood Cell	Red Blood Cell
Hemoglobin	Hematocrit
Platelets	Other

Questions to ask the doctor: _____

_____

_____

_____

_____

_____

_____

Doctor's Diagnosis/Feedback: _____

_____

_____

_____

_____

Treatment Received Today: _____

_____

_____

Any medication changes? _____

_____

_____

Office Visit

Next Visit

Date/Time _____

Purpose _____

Who will I see? _____

Today I'm feeling:

O   Better   O   Worse   O   Same

O   Pain   O   Fatigue   O   Depression

NOTES

Office Visit

Date/Time: _____

Doctor: _____

Reason for Visit: _____

Blood Cell Count

White Blood Cell	Red Blood Cell
Hemoglobin	Hematocrit
Platelets	Other

Questions to ask the doctor: _____
_____
_____
_____
_____
_____
_____

Doctor's Diagnosis/Feedback: _____
_____
_____
_____

Treatment Received Today: _____
_____
_____

Any medication changes? _____
_____
_____

Next Visit

Date/Time _____

Purpose _____

Who will I see? _____

Today I'm feeling:

    O   Better   O   Worse   O   Same

    O   Pain   O   Fatigue   O   Depression

NOTES

Office Visit

Date/Time: _____

Doctor: _____

Reason for Visit: _____

Blood Cell Count

White Blood Cell	Red Blood Cell
Hemoglobin	Hematocrit
Platelets	Other

Questions to ask the doctor: _____

_____

_____

_____

_____

_____

_____

Doctor's Diagnosis/Feedback: _____

_____

_____

_____

_____

Treatment Received Today: _____

_____

_____

Any medication changes? _____

_____

_____

Office Visit

Next Visit

Date/Time _____

Purpose _____

Who will I see? _____

Today I'm feeling:

O   Better   O   Worse   O   Same

O   Pain   O   Fatigue   O   Depression

NOTES

Office Visit

Date/Time: _____

Doctor: _____

Reason for Visit: _____

Blood Cell Count

White Blood Cell	Red Blood Cell
Hemoglobin	Hematocrit
Platelets	Other

Questions to ask the doctor: _____
_____
_____
_____
_____
_____
_____

Doctor's Diagnosis/Feedback: _____
_____
_____
_____
_____

Treatment Received Today: _____
_____
_____

Any medication changes? _____
_____
_____

Office Visit

Next Visit

Date/Time _____

Purpose _____

Who will I see? _____

Today I'm feeling:

O   Better   O   Worse   O   Same

O   Pain   O   Fatigue   O   Depression

NOTES

Office Visit

Date/Time: _____

Doctor: _____

Reason for Visit: _____

Blood Cell Count

White Blood Cell	Red Blood Cell
Hemoglobin	Hematocrit
Platelets	Other

Questions to ask the doctor: _____
_____
_____
_____
_____
_____
_____

Doctor's Diagnosis/Feedback: _____
_____
_____
_____
_____

Treatment Received Today: _____
_____
_____

Any medication changes? _____
_____
_____

Next Visit

Date/Time _____

Purpose _____

Who will I see? _____

Today I'm feeling:

    O   Better   O   Worse   O   Same

    O   Pain   O   Fatigue   O   Depression

NOTES

Office Visit

Date/Time: _____

Doctor: _____

Reason for Visit: _____

Blood Cell Count

White Blood Cell	Red Blood Cell
Hemoglobin	Hematocrit
Platelets	Other

Questions to ask the doctor: _____
_____
_____
_____
_____
_____
_____

Doctor's Diagnosis/Feedback: _____
_____
_____
_____
_____

Treatment Received Today: _____
_____
_____

Any medication changes? _____
_____
_____

Next Visit

Date/Time _____

Purpose _____

Who will I see? _____

Today I'm feeling:

O Better   O Worse   O Same

O Pain   O Fatigue   O Depression

NOTES

Office Visit

Date/Time: _____

Doctor: _____

Reason for Visit: _____

Blood Cell Count

White Blood Cell	Red Blood Cell
Hemoglobin	Hematocrit
Platelets	Other

Questions to ask the doctor: _____
_____
_____
_____
_____
_____
_____

Doctor's Diagnosis/Feedback: _____
_____
_____
_____
_____

Treatment Received Today: _____
_____
_____

Any medication changes? _____
_____
_____

Next Visit

Date/Time _____

Purpose _____

Who will I see? _____

Today I'm feeling:

O   Better   O   Worse   O   Same

O   Pain   O   Fatigue   O   Depression

NOTES

Office Visit

Date/Time: _____

Doctor: _____

Reason for Visit: _____

Blood Cell Count

White Blood Cell	Red Blood Cell
Hemoglobin	Hematocrit
Platelets	Other

Questions to ask the doctor: _____

_____

_____

_____

_____

_____

_____

Doctor's Diagnosis/Feedback: _____

_____

_____

_____

_____

Treatment Received Today: _____

_____

_____

Any medication changes? _____

_____

_____

Next Visit

Date/Time _____

Purpose _____

Who will I see? _____

Today I'm feeling:

O   Better   O   Worse   O   Same

O   Pain   O   Fatigue   O   Depression

NOTES

Office Visit

Date/Time: _____

Doctor: _____

Reason for Visit: _____

Blood Cell Count

White Blood Cell	Red Blood Cell
Hemoglobin	Hematocrit
Platelets	Other

Questions to ask the doctor: _____

_____

_____

_____

_____

_____

_____

Doctor's Diagnosis/Feedback: _____

_____

_____

_____

_____

Treatment Received Today: _____

_____

_____

Any medication changes? _____

_____

_____

Next Visit

Date/Time _____

Purpose _____

Who will I see? _____

Today I'm feeling:

    O   Better   O   Worse   O   Same

    O   Pain   O   Fatigue   O   Depression

NOTES

Office Visit

Date/Time: _____

Doctor: _____

Reason for Visit: _____

Blood Cell Count

White Blood Cell	Red Blood Cell
Hemoglobin	Hematocrit
Platelets	Other

Questions to ask the doctor: _____

_____
_____
_____
_____
_____
_____

Doctor's Diagnosis/Feedback: _____

_____
_____
_____
_____

Treatment Received Today: _____

_____
_____

Any medication changes? _____

_____
_____

Next Visit

Date/Time _____

Purpose _____

Who will I see? _____

Today I'm feeling:

O Better	O Worse	O Same
O Pain	O Fatigue	O Depression

NOTES

Office Visit

Date/Time: _____

Doctor: _____

Reason for Visit: _____

Blood Cell Count

White Blood Cell	Red Blood Cell
Hemoglobin	Hematocrit
Platelets	Other

Questions to ask the doctor: _____
_____
_____
_____
_____
_____
_____

Doctor's Diagnosis/Feedback: _____
_____
_____
_____
_____

Treatment Received Today: _____
_____
_____

Any medication changes? _____
_____
_____

Next Visit

Date/Time _____

Purpose _____

Who will I see? _____

Today I'm feeling:

    O   Better   O   Worse   O   Same

    O   Pain   O   Fatigue   O   Depression

NOTES

Office Visit

Date/Time: _____

Doctor: _____

Reason for Visit: _____

Blood Cell Count

White Blood Cell	Red Blood Cell
Hemoglobin	Hematocrit
Platelets	Other

Questions to ask the doctor: _____

_____

_____

_____

_____

_____

_____

Doctor's Diagnosis/Feedback: _____

_____

_____

_____

_____

Treatment Received Today: _____

_____

_____

Any medication changes? _____

_____

_____

Next Visit

Date/Time _____

Purpose _____

Who will I see? _____

Today I'm feeling:

- O   Better
- O   Worse
- O   Same
- O   Pain
- O   Fatigue
- O   Depression

NOTES

Office Visit

Date/Time: _____

Doctor: _____

Reason for Visit: _____

Blood Cell Count

White Blood Cell	Red Blood Cell
Hemoglobin	Hematocrit
Platelets	Other

Questions to ask the doctor: _____

_____
_____
_____
_____
_____
_____

Doctor's Diagnosis/Feedback: _____

_____
_____
_____
_____

Treatment Received Today: _____

_____
_____

Any medication changes? _____

_____
_____

Next Visit

Date/Time _____

Purpose _____

Who will I see? _____

Today I'm feeling:

    O   Better   O   Worse   O   Same

    O   Pain   O   Fatigue   O   Depression

NOTES

Office Visit

Date/Time: _____

Doctor: _____

Reason for Visit: _____

Blood Cell Count

White Blood Cell	Red Blood Cell
Hemoglobin	Hematocrit
Platelets	Other

Questions to ask the doctor: _____
_____
_____
_____
_____
_____
_____

Doctor's Diagnosis/Feedback: _____
_____
_____
_____
_____

Treatment Received Today: _____
_____
_____

Any medication changes? _____
_____
_____

Office Visit

Next Visit

Date/Time _____

Purpose _____

Who will I see? _____

Today I'm feeling:

    O   Better   O   Worse   O   Same

    O   Pain   O   Fatigue   O   Depression

NOTES

Office Visit

Date/Time: _____

Doctor: _____

Reason for Visit: _____

Blood Cell Count

White Blood Cell	Red Blood Cell
Hemoglobin	Hematocrit
Platelets	Other

Questions to ask the doctor: _____
_____
_____
_____
_____
_____
_____

Doctor's Diagnosis/Feedback: _____
_____
_____
_____
_____

Treatment Received Today: _____
_____
_____

Any medication changes? _____
_____
_____

Next Visit

Date/Time _____

Purpose _____

Who will I see? _____

Today I'm feeling:

○   Better   ○   Worse   ○   Same

○   Pain   ○   Fatigue   ○   Depression

NOTES

Office Visit

Date/Time: _____

Doctor: _____

Reason for Visit: _____

Blood Cell Count

White Blood Cell	Red Blood Cell
Hemoglobin	Hematocrit
Platelets	Other

Questions to ask the doctor: _____
_____
_____
_____
_____
_____
_____

Doctor's Diagnosis/Feedback: _____
_____
_____
_____
_____

Treatment Received Today: _____
_____
_____

Any medication changes? _____
_____
_____

Next Visit

Date/Time _____

Purpose _____

Who will I see? _____

Today I'm feeling:

  O Better   O Worse   O Same

  O Pain   O Fatigue   O Depression

NOTES

Office Visit

Date/Time: _____

Doctor: _____

Reason for Visit: _____

Blood Cell Count

White Blood Cell	Red Blood Cell
Hemoglobin	Hematocrit
Platelets	Other

Questions to ask the doctor: _____
_____
_____
_____
_____
_____
_____

Doctor's Diagnosis/Feedback: _____
_____
_____
_____
_____

Treatment Received Today: _____
_____
_____

Any medication changes? _____
_____
_____

Next Visit

Date/Time _____

Purpose _____

Who will I see? _____

Today I'm feeling:

    O   Better   O   Worse   O   Same

    O   Pain   O   Fatigue   O   Depression

NOTES

My Journal

Week of _____

Monday

Tuesday

Wednesday

Thursday

My Journal

Friday

Saturday

Sunday

Notes

My Journal

Week of _____

Monday

Tuesday

Wednesday

Thursday

My Journal

Friday

Saturday

Sunday

Notes

My Journal

Week of _____

Monday

Tuesday

Wednesday

Thursday

My Journal

Friday

Saturday

Sunday

Notes

My Journal

Week of _____

Monday

Tuesday

Wednesday

Thursday

My Journal

Friday

Saturday

Sunday

Notes

My Journal

Week of _____

Monday

Tuesday

Wednesday

Thursday

My Journal

Friday

Saturday

Sunday

Notes

My Journal

Week of _____

Monday

Tuesday

Wednesday

Thursday

My Journal

Friday

Saturday

Sunday

Notes

My Journal

Week of _____

Monday

Tuesday

Wednesday

Thursday

My Journal

Friday

Saturday

Sunday

Notes

My Journal

Week of _____

Monday

Tuesday

Wednesday

Thursday

My Journal

Friday

Saturday

Sunday

Notes

My Journal

Week of _____

Monday

Tuesday

Wednesday

Thursday

My Journal

Friday

Saturday

Sunday

Notes

My Journal

Week of _____

Monday

Tuesday

Wednesday

Thursday

My Journal

Friday

Saturday

Sunday

Notes

My Journal

Week of _____

Monday

Tuesday

Wednesday

Thursday

My Journal

Friday

Saturday

Sunday

Notes

My Journal

Week of _____

Monday

Tuesday

Wednesday

Thursday

My Journal

Friday

Saturday

Sunday

Notes

My Journal

Week of _____

Monday

Tuesday

Wednesday

Thursday

My Journal

Friday

Saturday

Sunday

Notes

My Journal

Week of _____

Monday

Tuesday

Wednesday

Thursday

My Journal

Friday

Saturday

Sunday

Notes

My Journal

Week of _____

Monday

Tuesday

Wednesday

Thursday

My Journal

Friday

Saturday

Sunday

Notes

My Journal

Week of _____

Monday

Tuesday

Wednesday

Thursday

My Journal

Friday

Saturday

Sunday

Notes

My Journal

Week of _____

Monday

Tuesday

Wednesday

Thursday

My Journal

Friday

Saturday

Sunday

Notes

My Journal

Week of _____

Monday

Tuesday

Wednesday

Thursday

My Journal

Friday

Saturday

Sunday

Notes

My Journal

Week of _____

Monday

Tuesday

Wednesday

Thursday

My Journal

Friday

Saturday

Sunday

Notes

My Journal

Week of _____

Monday

Tuesday

Wednesday

Thursday

My Journal

Friday

Saturday

Sunday

Notes

My Journal

week of _____

Monday

Tuesday

Wednesday

Thursday

My Journal

Friday

Saturday

Sunday

Notes

My Journal

Week of _____

Monday

Tuesday

Wednesday

Thursday

My Journal

Friday

Saturday

Sunday

Notes

My Journal

Week of _____

Monday

Tuesday

Wednesday

Thursday

My Journal

Friday

Saturday

Sunday

Notes

My Journal

Week of _____

Monday

Tuesday

Wednesday

Thursday

My Journal

Friday

Saturday

Sunday

Notes

My Journal

Week of _____

Monday

Tuesday

Wednesday

Thursday

My Journal

Friday

Saturday

Sunday

Notes

My Journal

Week of _____

Monday

Tuesday

Wednesday

Thursday

My Journal

Friday

Saturday

Sunday

Notes

My Journal

Week of _____

Monday

Tuesday

Wednesday

Thursday

My Journal

Friday

Saturday

Sunday

Notes

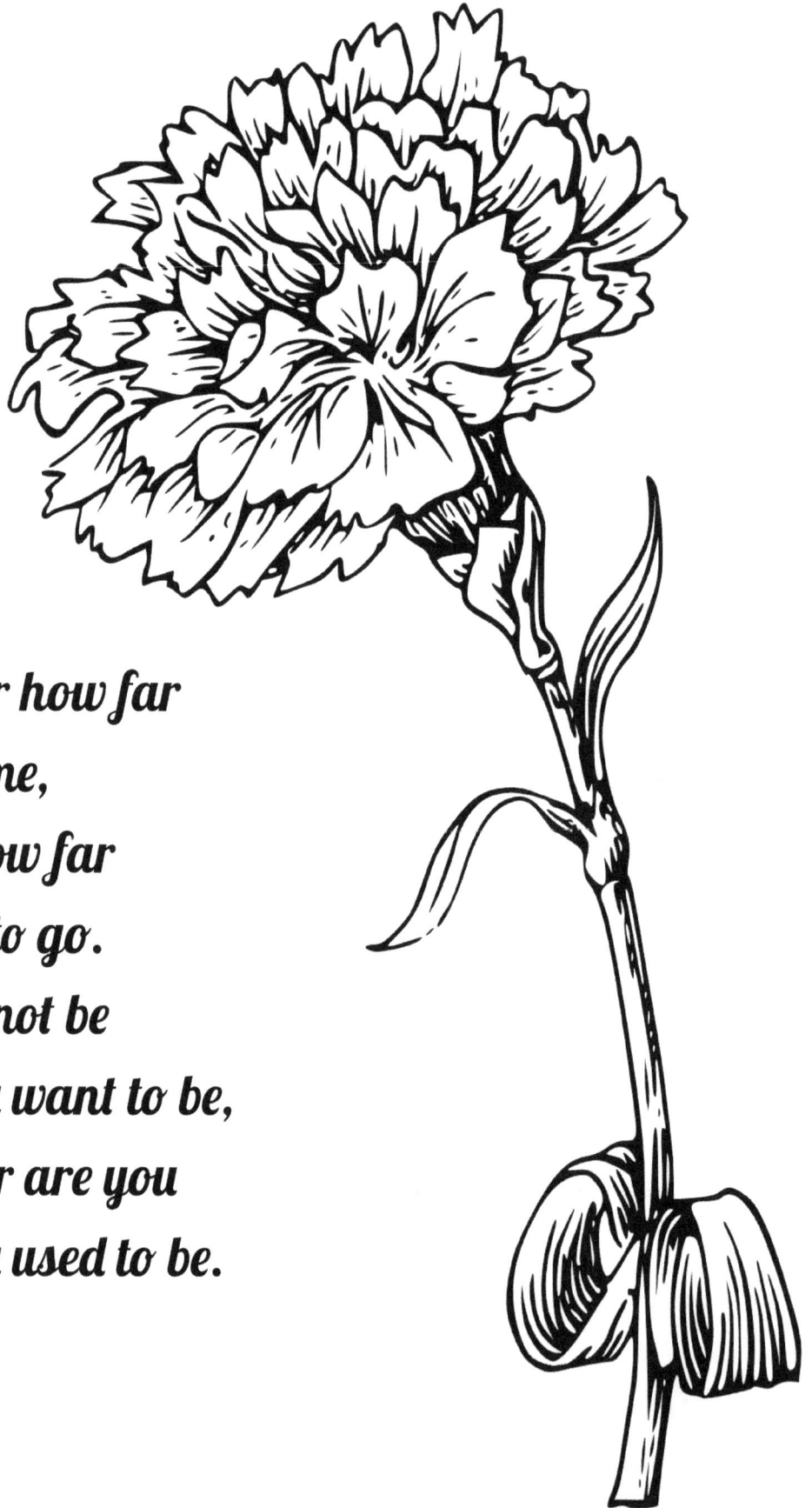

Remember how far
you've come,
not just how far
you have to go.
You may not be
where you want to be,
but neither are you
where you used to be.

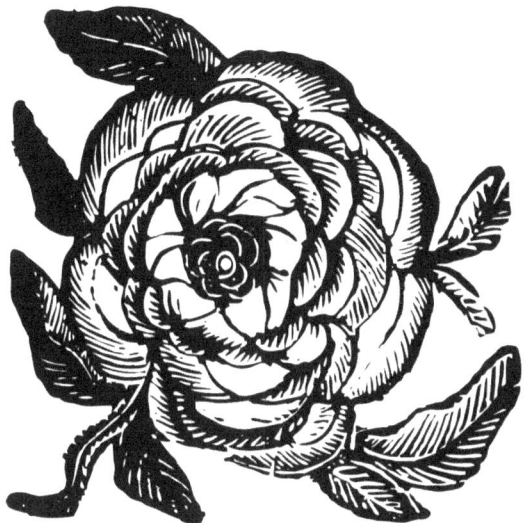

Above all, cancer is a spiritual practice that teaches me about faith and resilience.

— *Kris Carr*

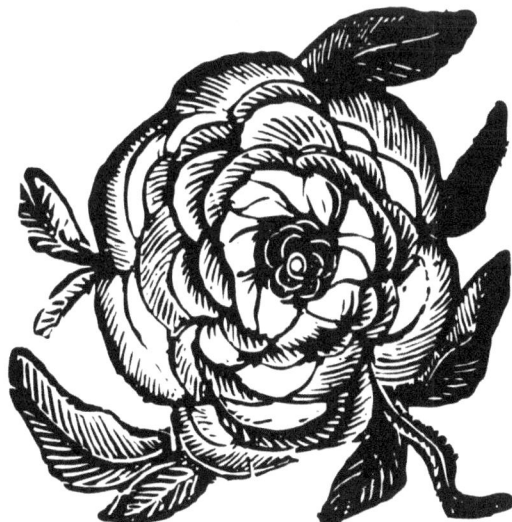

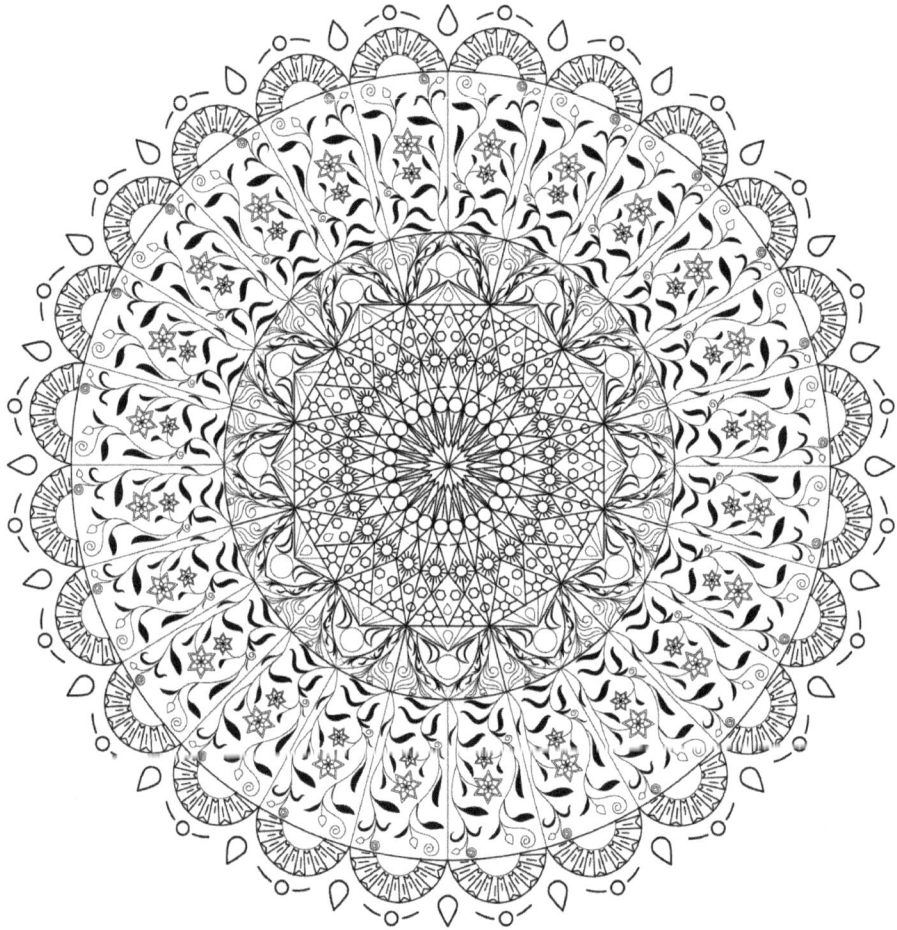

You know, once you've stood up to cancer, everything else feels like a pretty easy fight.

– David H. Koch

I think cancer is a hard battle to fight alone or with another person at your side, but I will say having someone to pick you up when you fall, stand by your side through every appointment and delivery of bad news, is priceless.

— Jenna Morasca

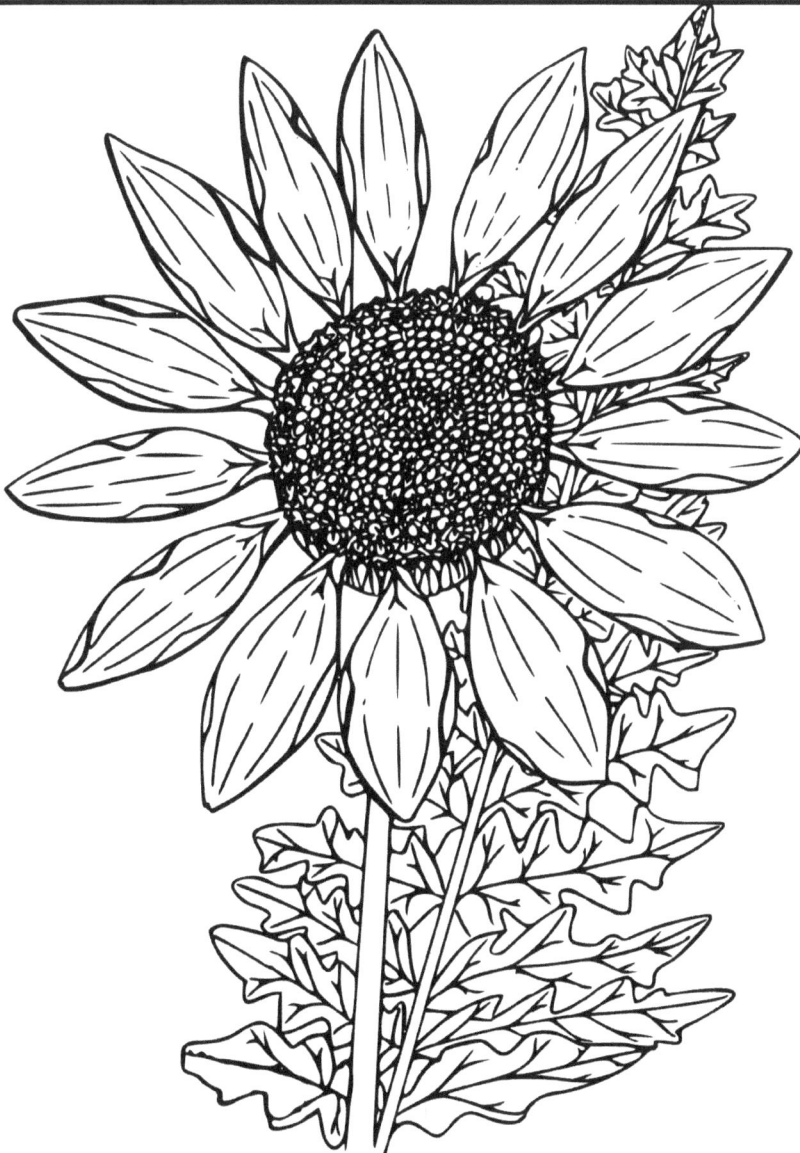

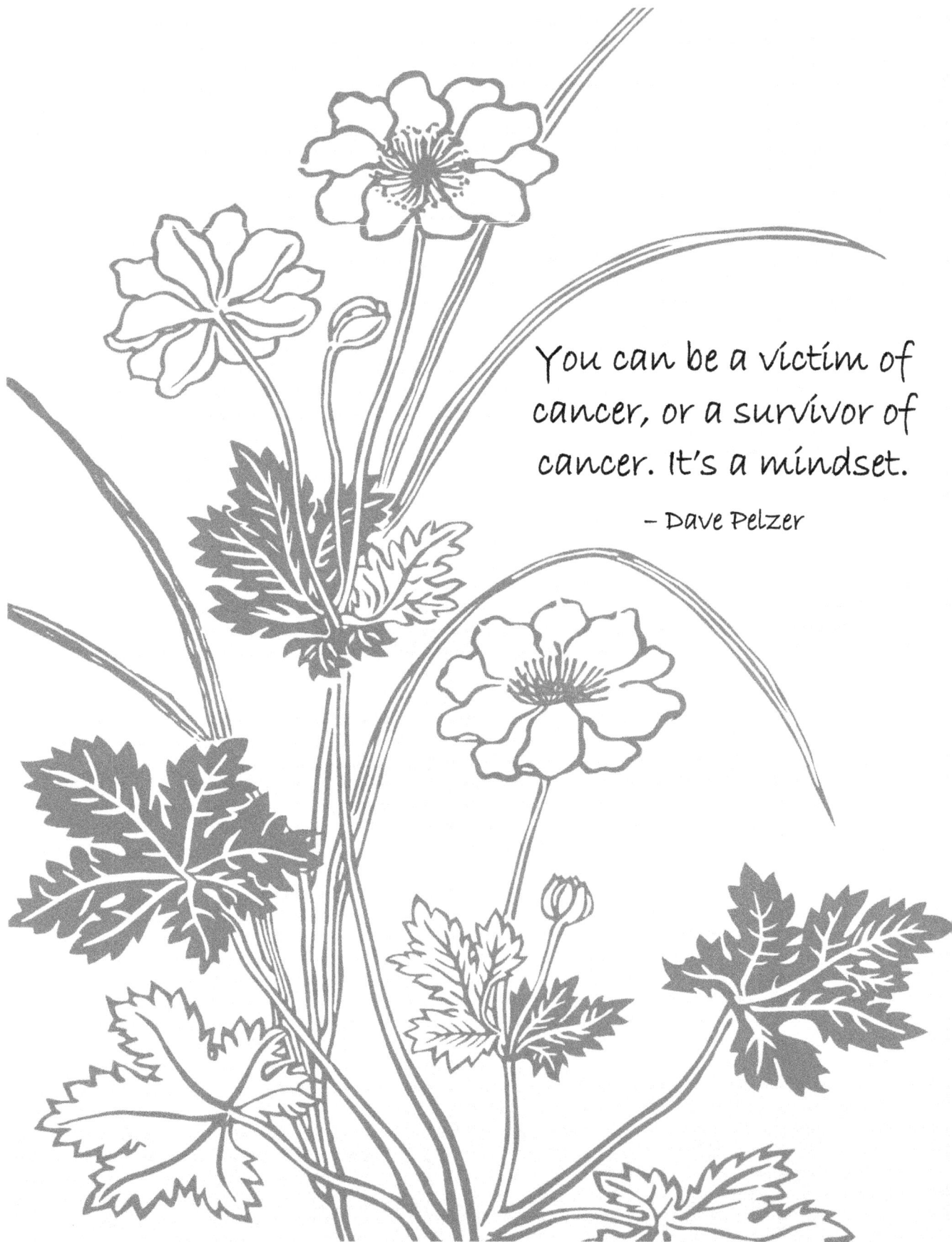

You can be a victim of cancer, or a survivor of cancer. It's a mindset.

– Dave Pelzer

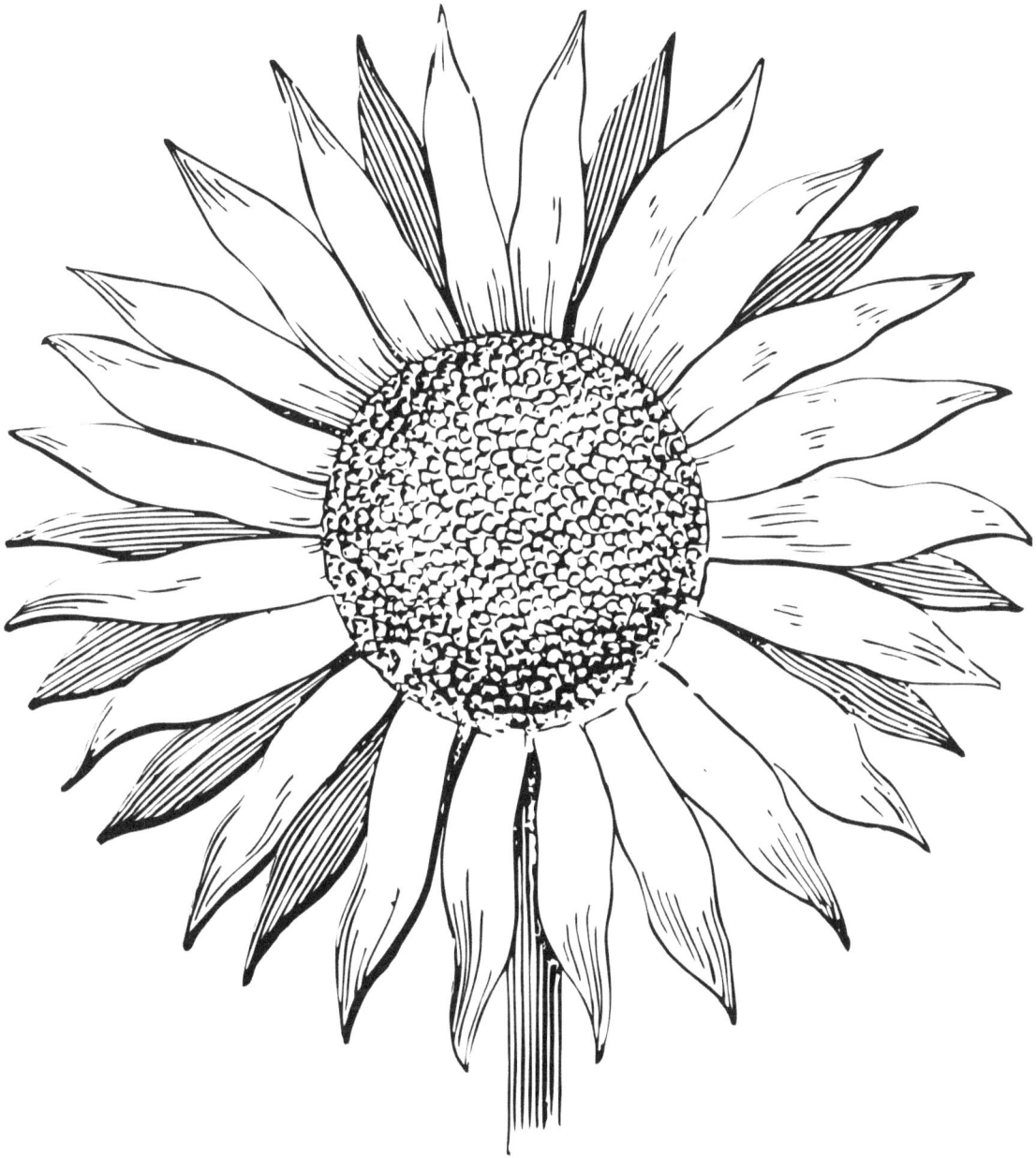

You are braver than you believe, stronger than you seem, smarter than you think, and twice as beautiful as you'd ever imagined.

We have two options, medically and emotionally: give up or fight like hell.

- Lance Armstrong

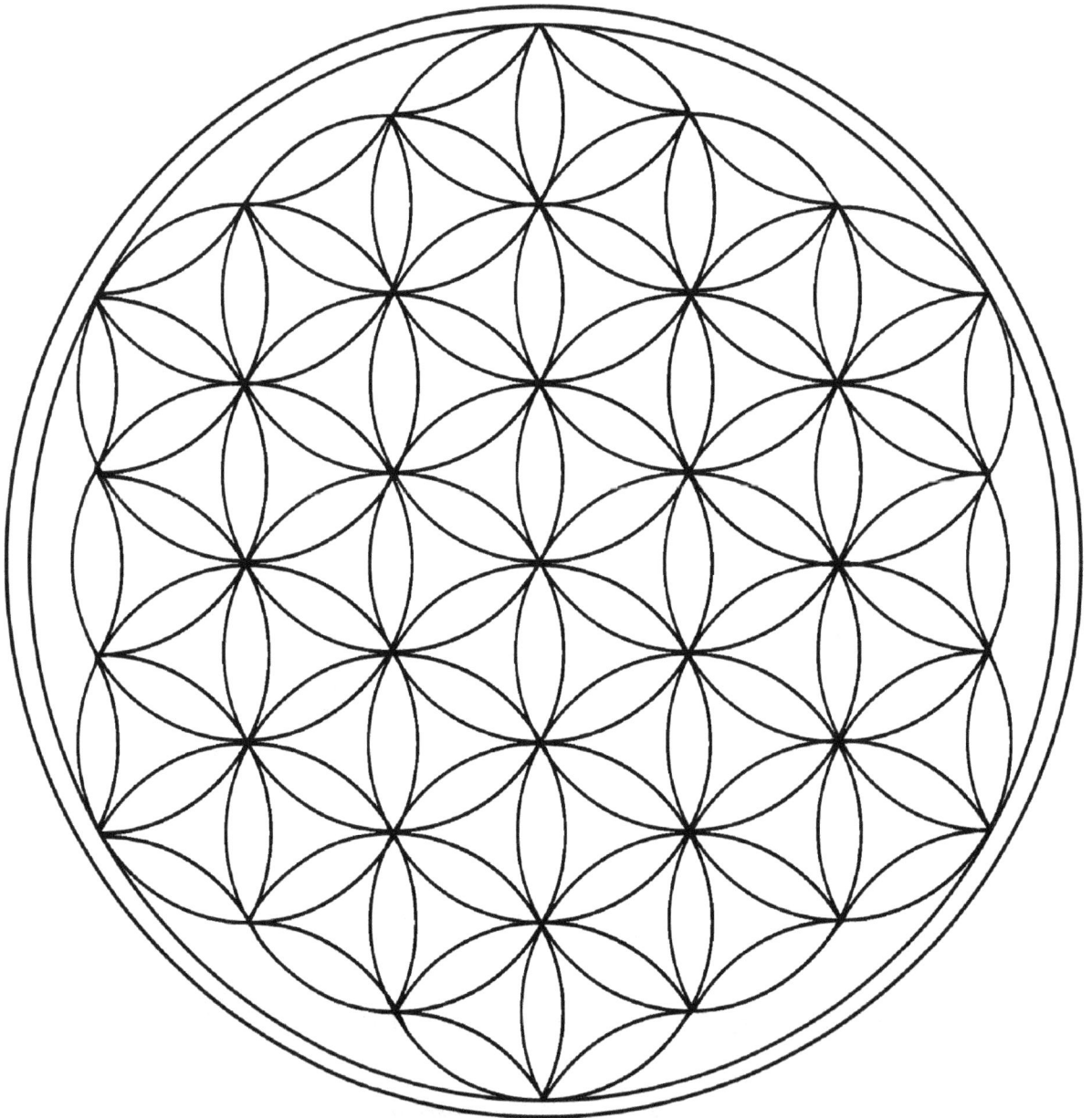

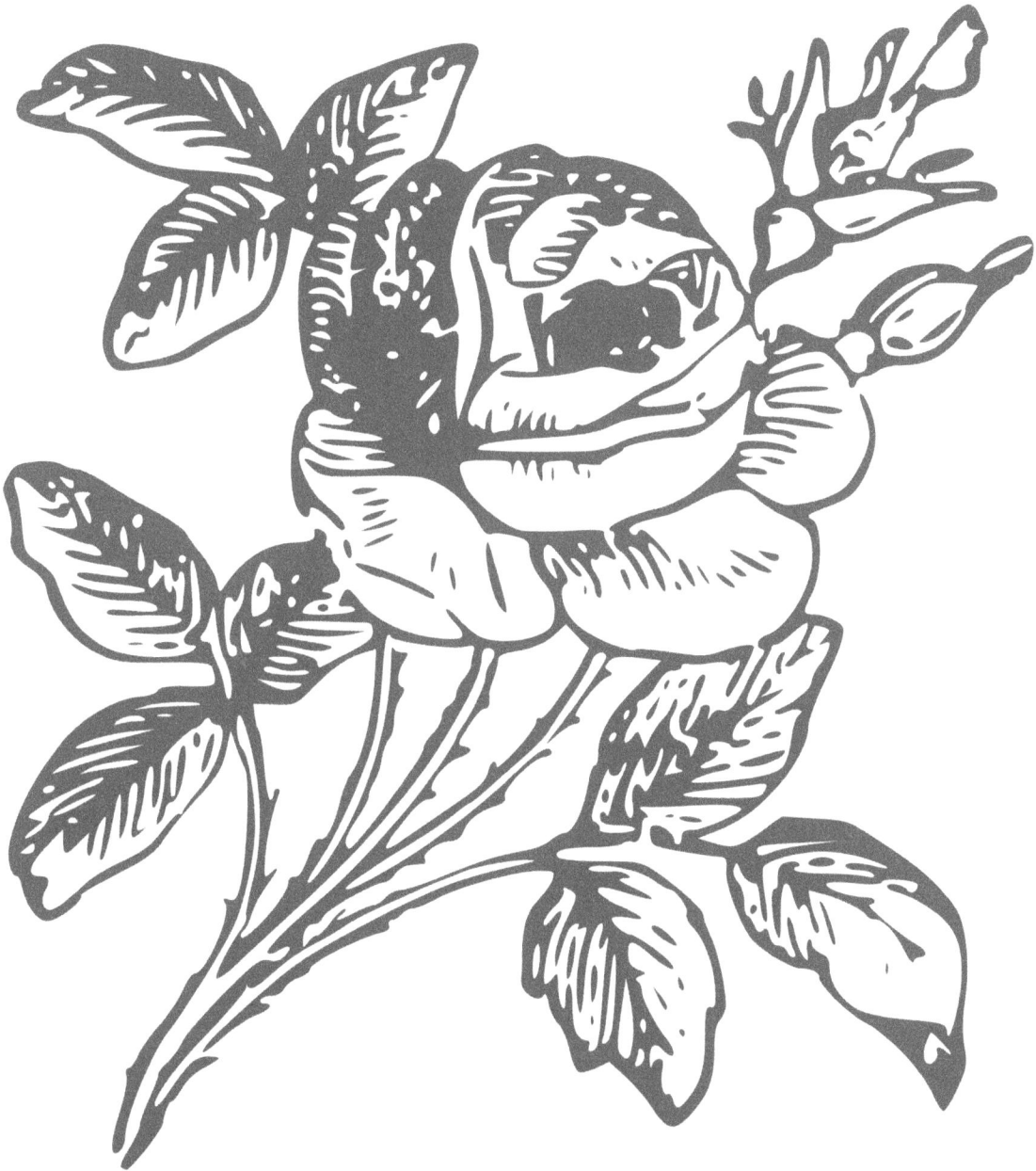

You never know how strong you are until being strong is the only choice you have.

– Cayla Mills

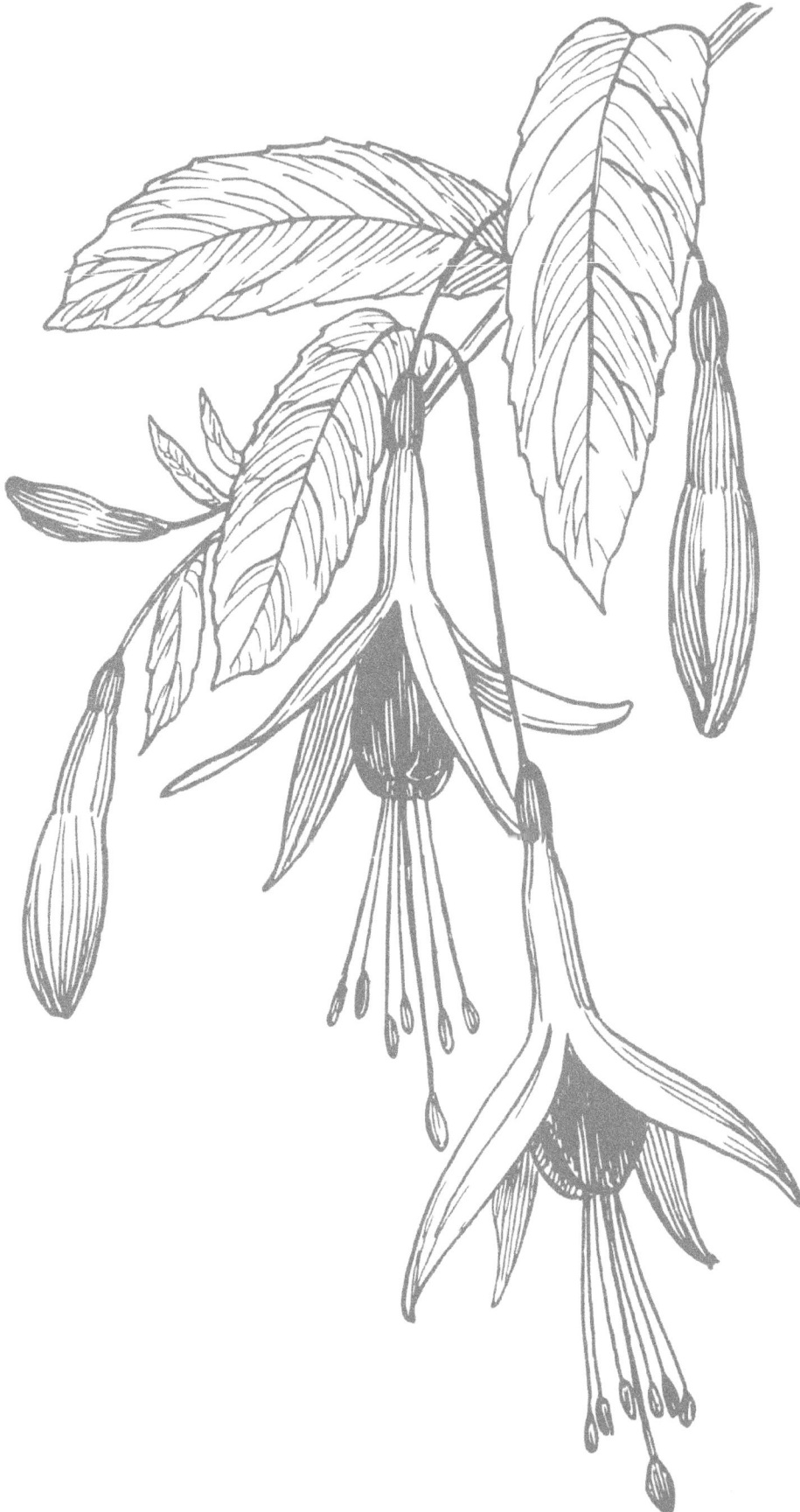

Be

thankful

for

this

day.

Small steps
every day.

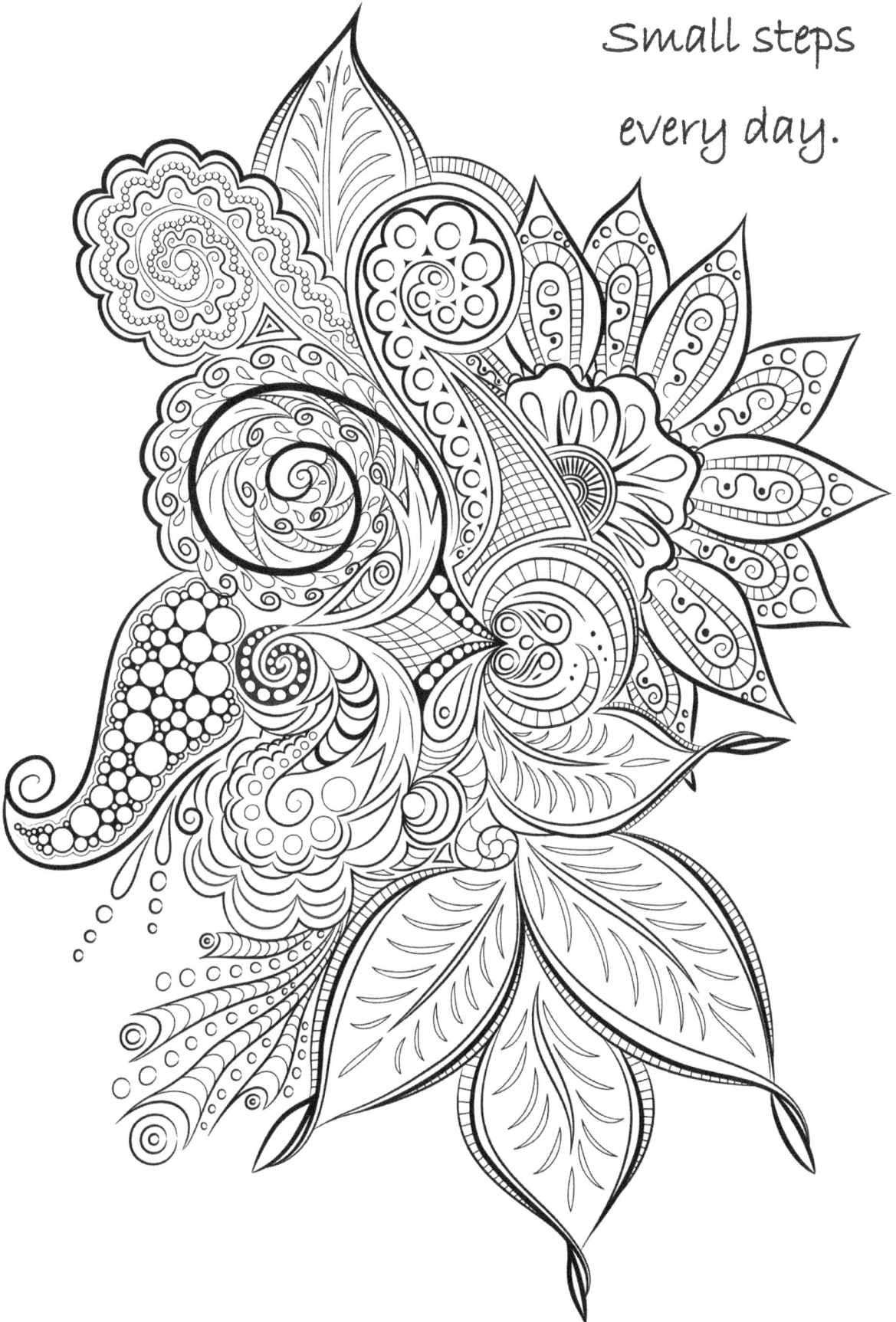

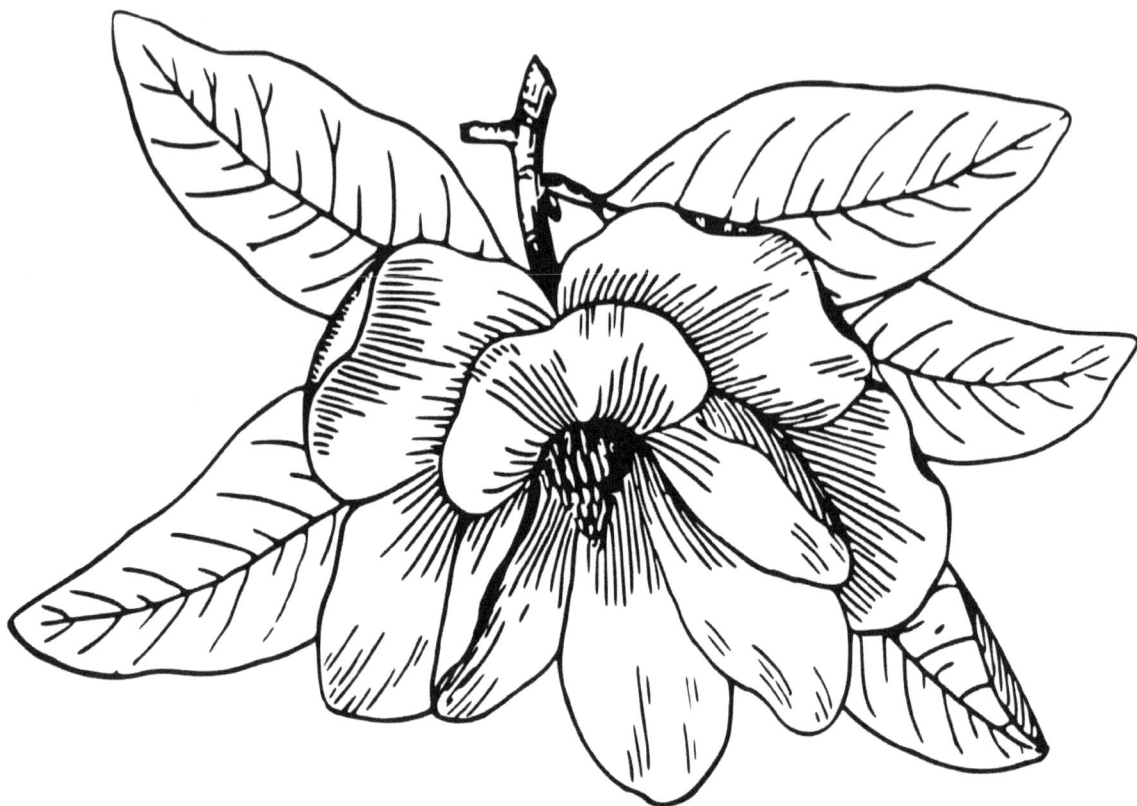

You beat cancer by how you
live, why you live and in the
manner in which you live.

– Stuart Scott

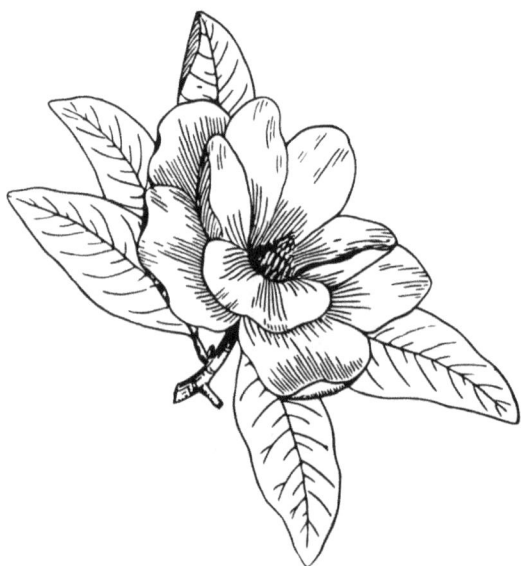

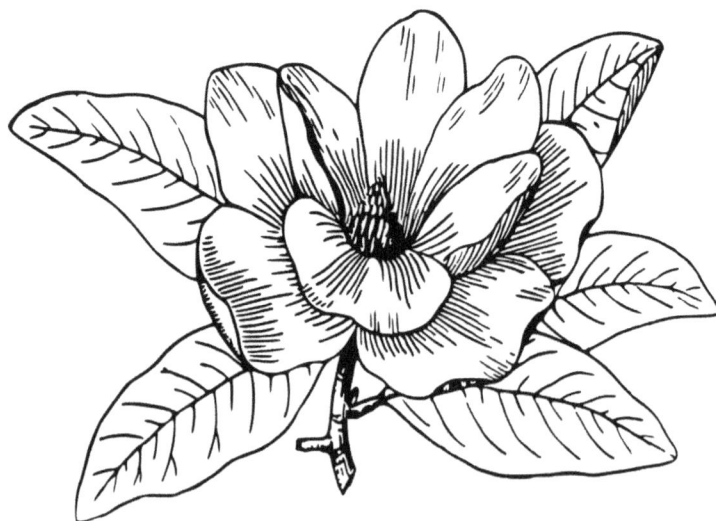

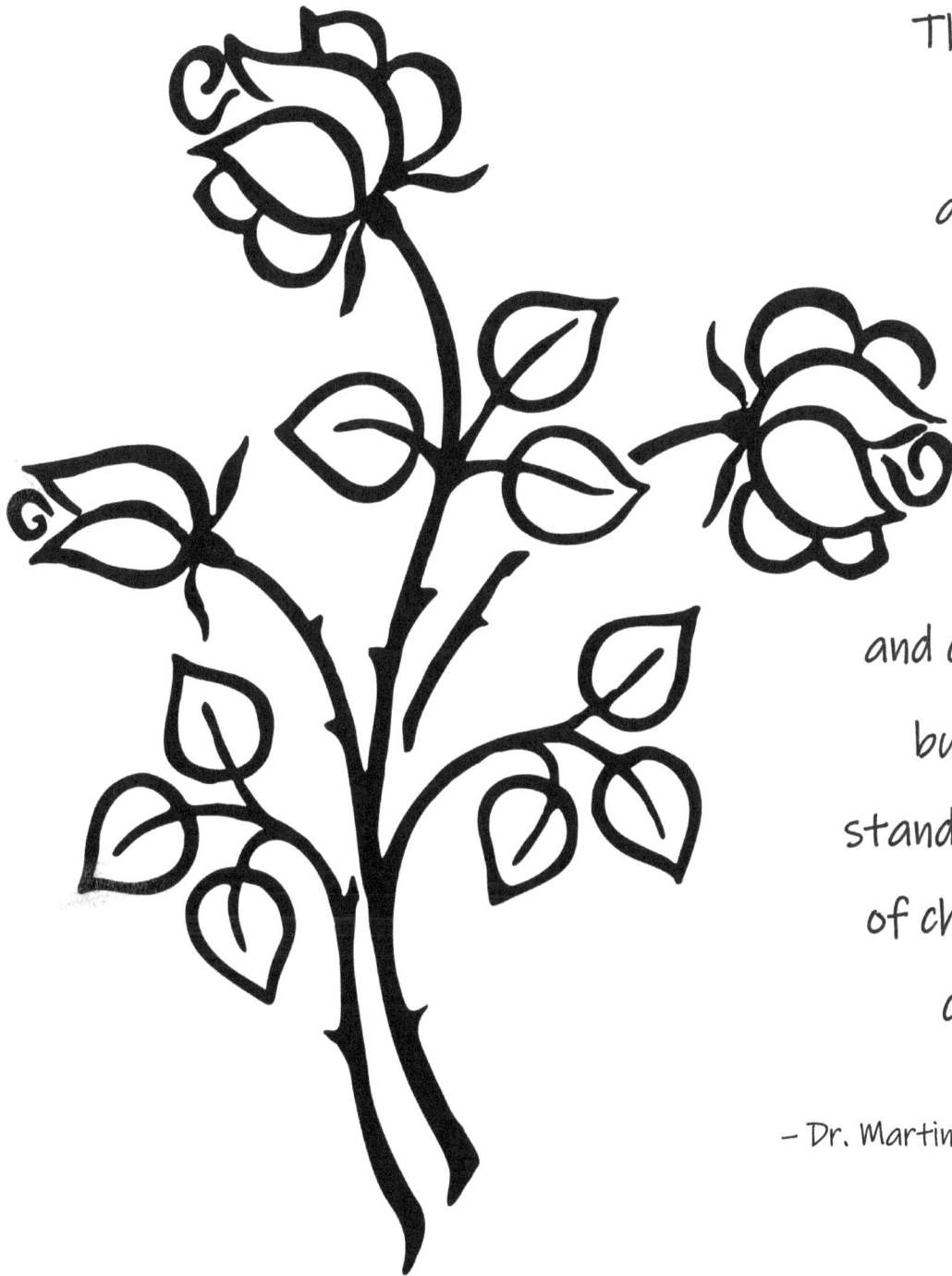

The ultimate
measure of
a man is not
where he
stands in
moments
of comfort
and convenience,
but where he
stands at a time
of challenge and
controversy.

– Dr. Martin Luther King Jr.

You gain strength, courage, and confidence by every experience in which you really stop to look fear in the face.

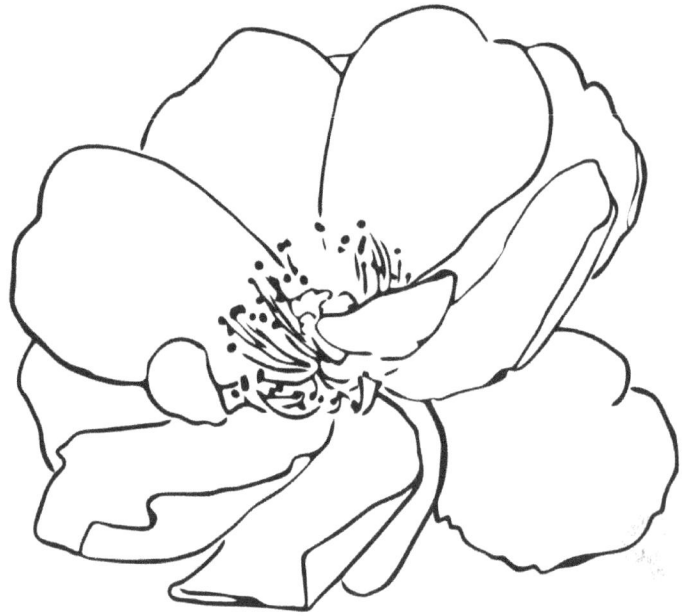

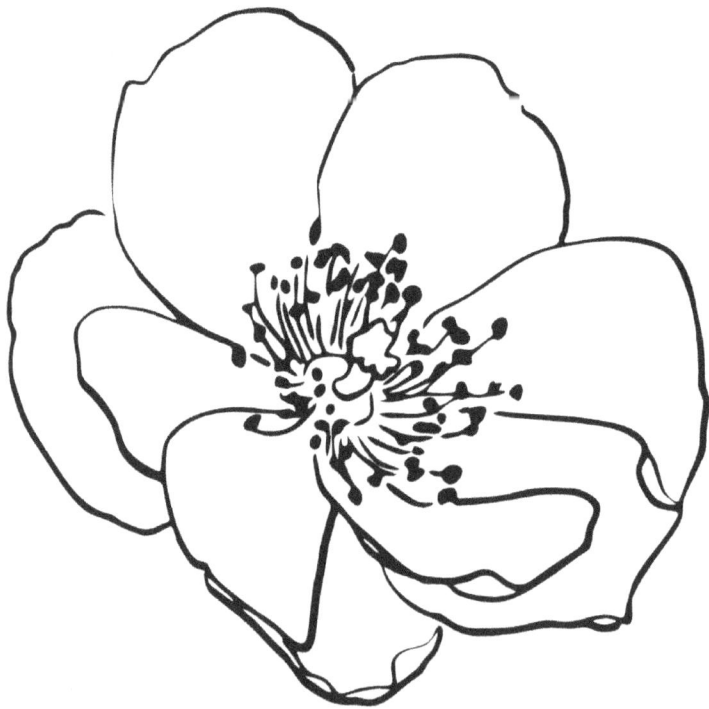

You must do the thing which you think you cannot do.

– Eleanor Roosevelt

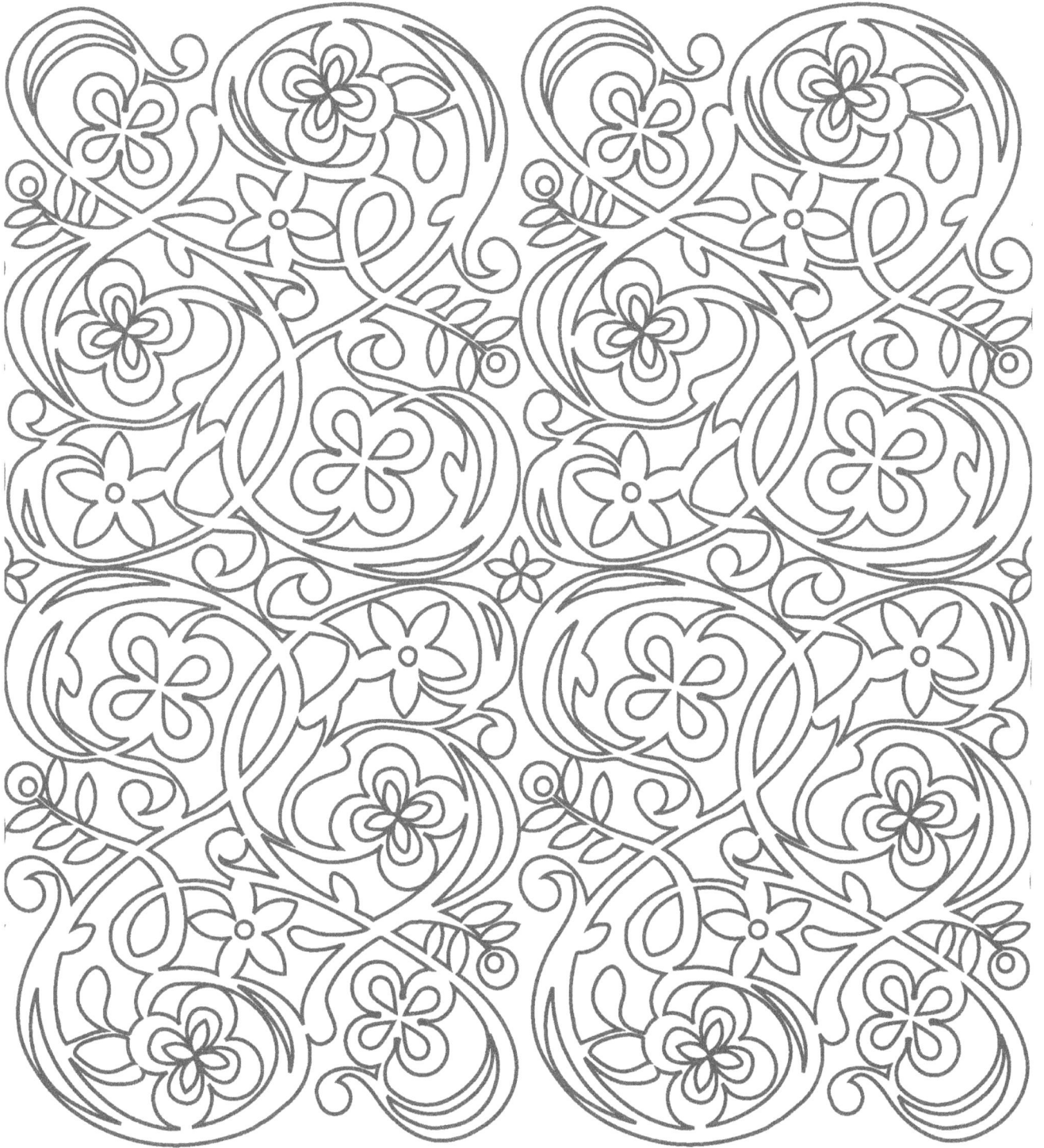

Never be ashamed of a scar. It simply means you were stronger than whatever tried to hurt you.

Cancer can take away all of my physical
abilities. It cannot touch my mind,

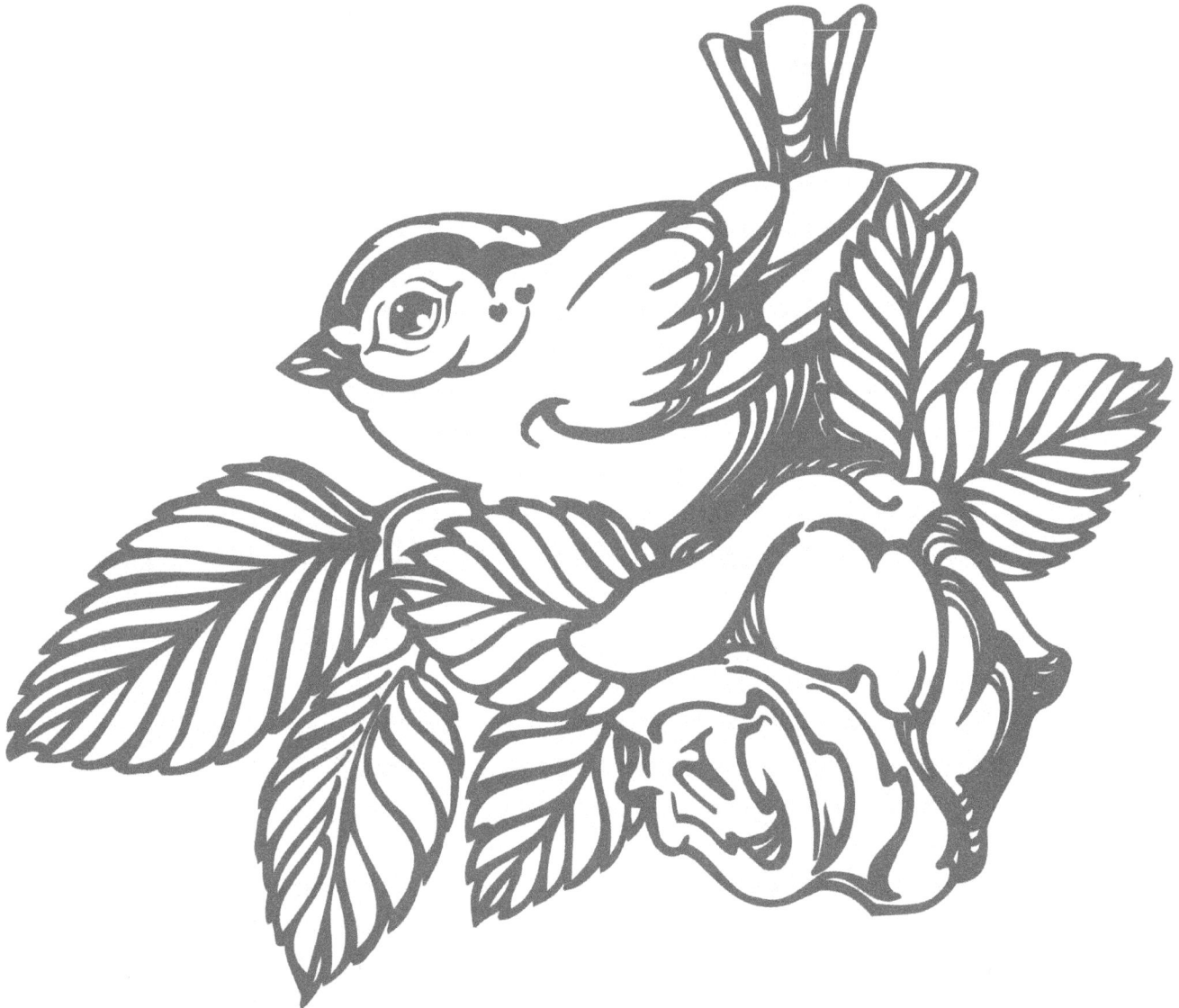

it cannot touch my heart,
and it cannot touch my soul.

- Jim Valvano

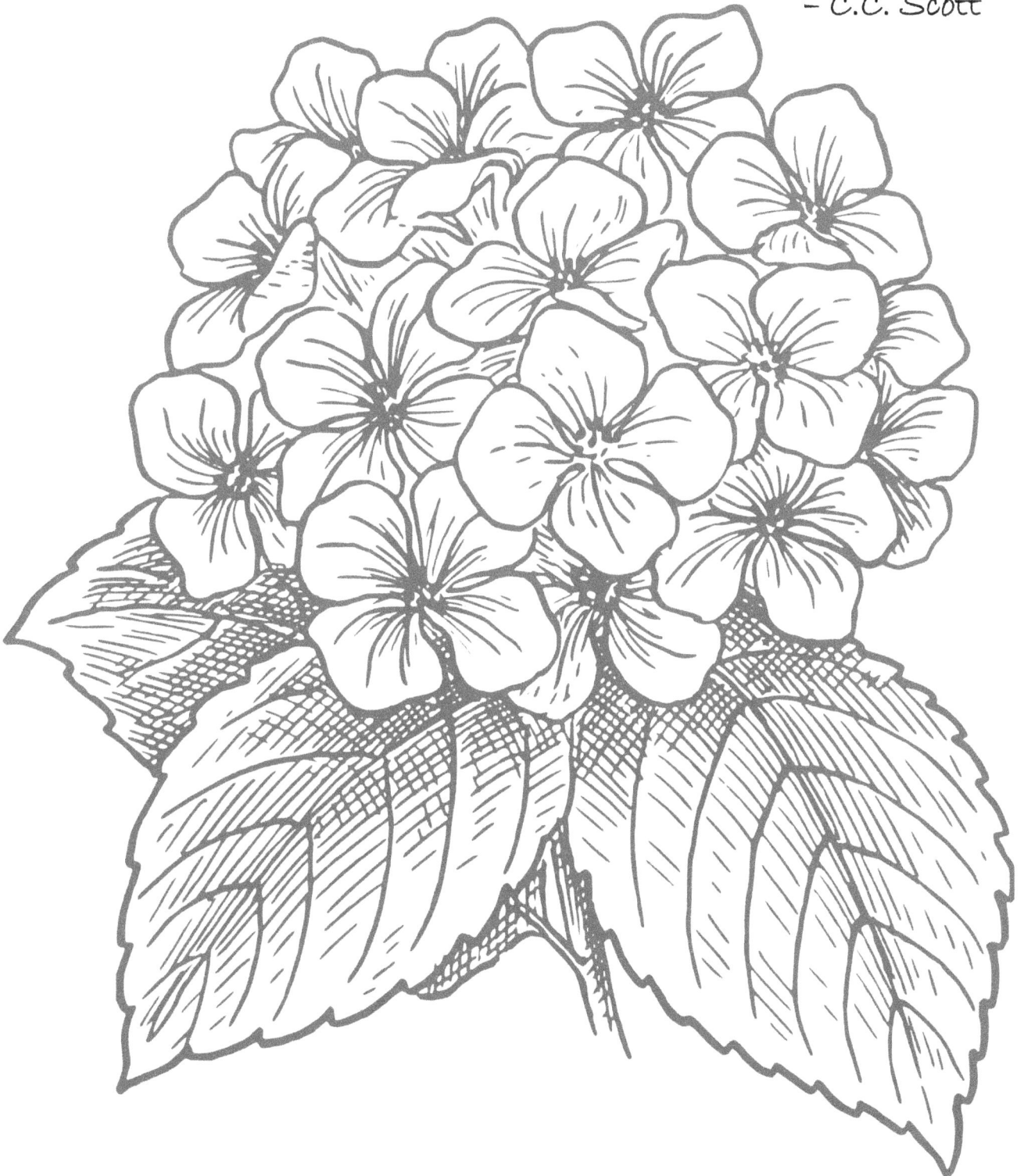

The human spirit is stronger than anything that can happen to it.

– C.C. Scott

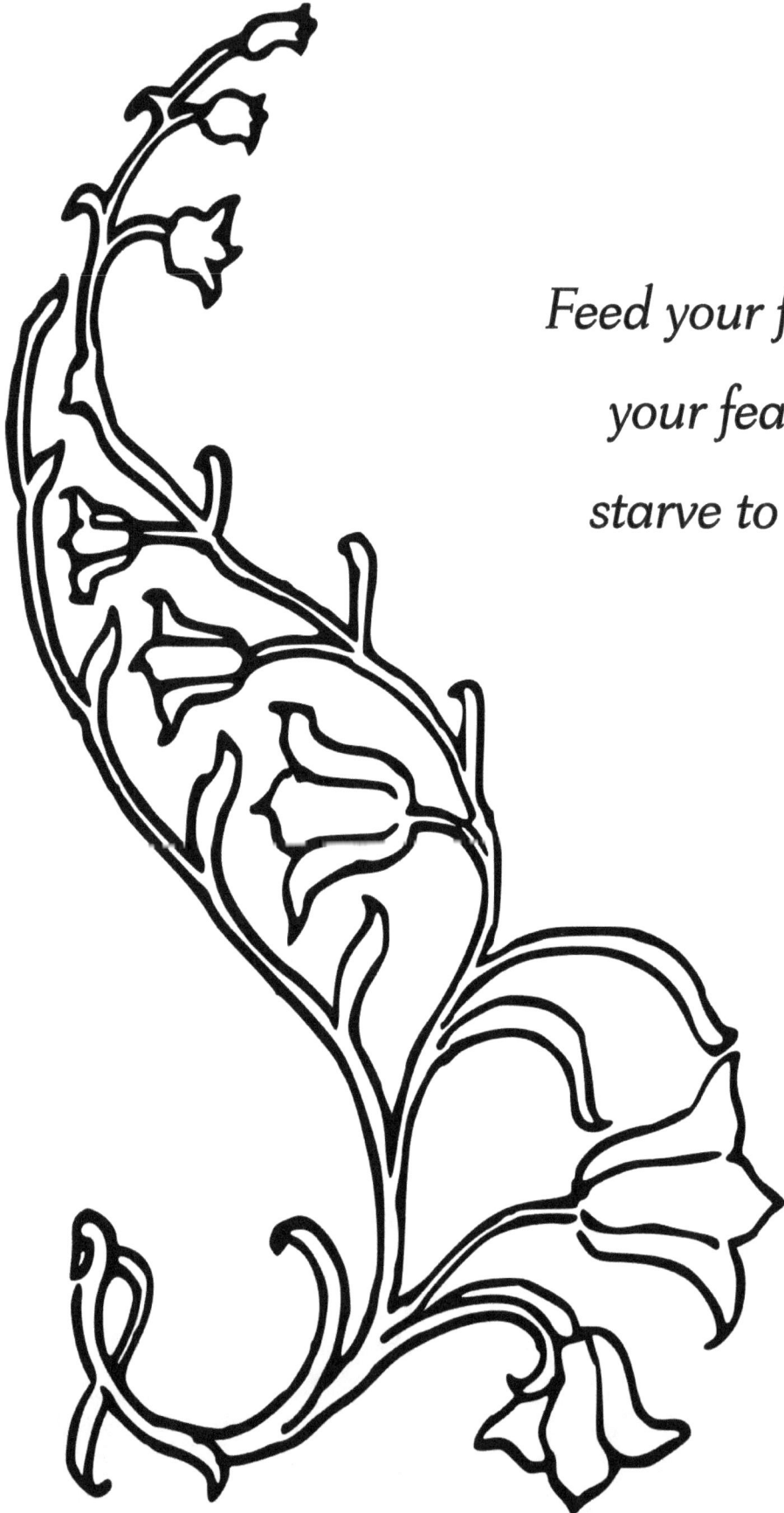

Feed your faith and

your fears will

starve to death.

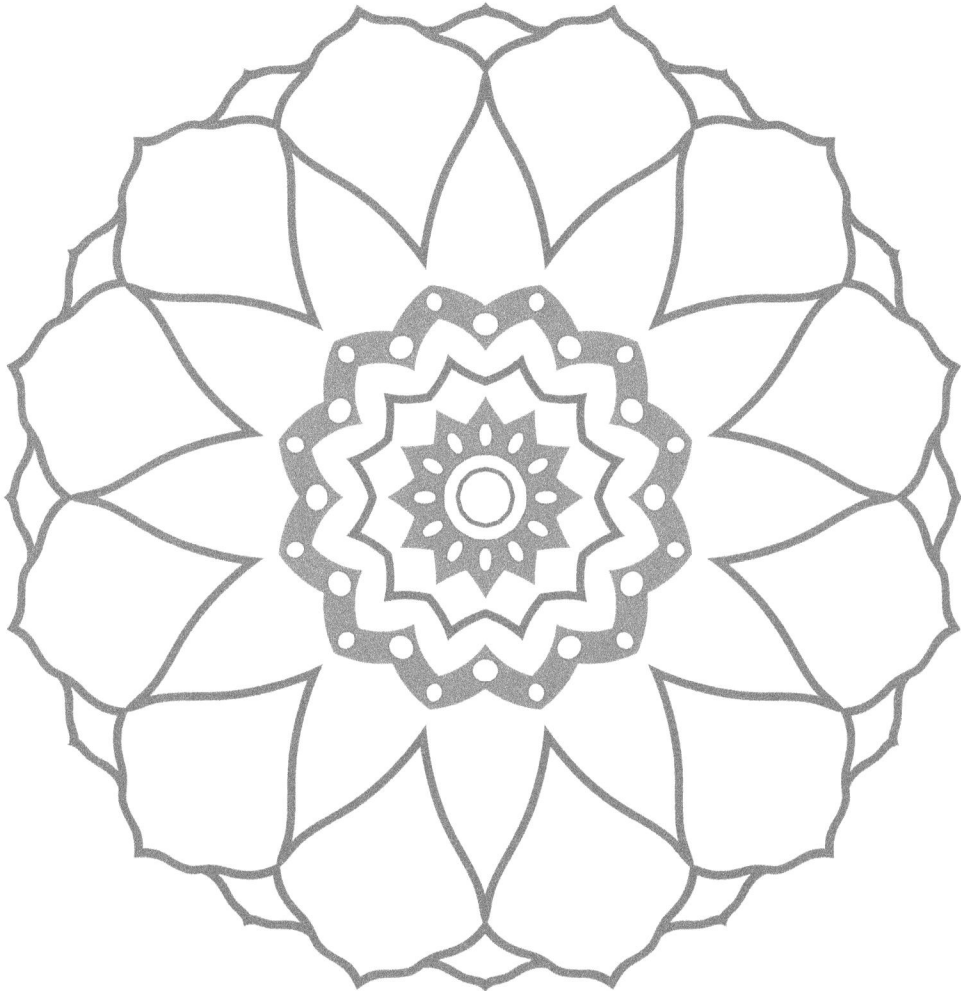

CANCER OPENS MANY DOORS.

ONE OF THE MOST

IMPORTANT IS YOUR HEART.

– Greg Anderson

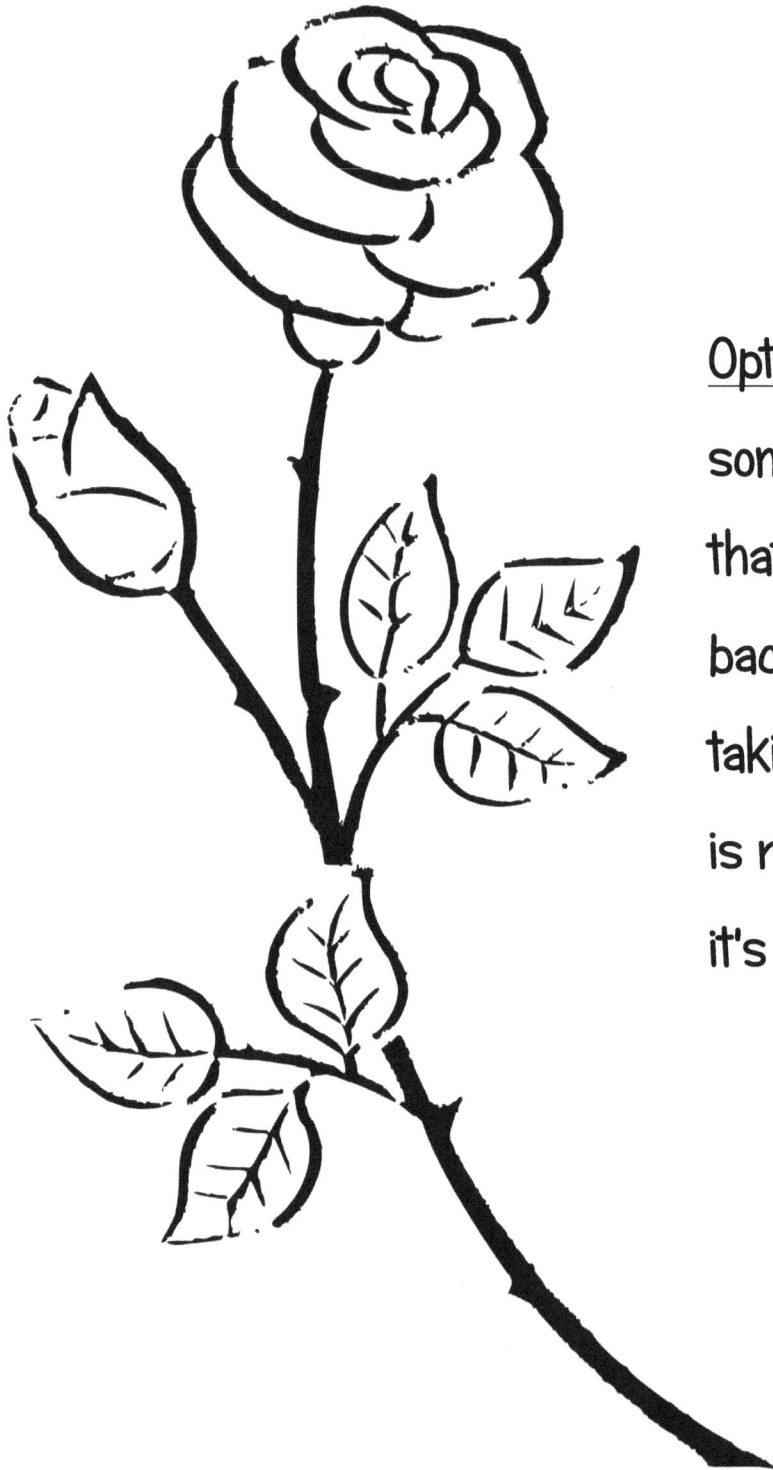

Optimism:

someone who figures

that taking a step

backward after

taking a step forward

is not a disaster;

it's more like a cha-cha.

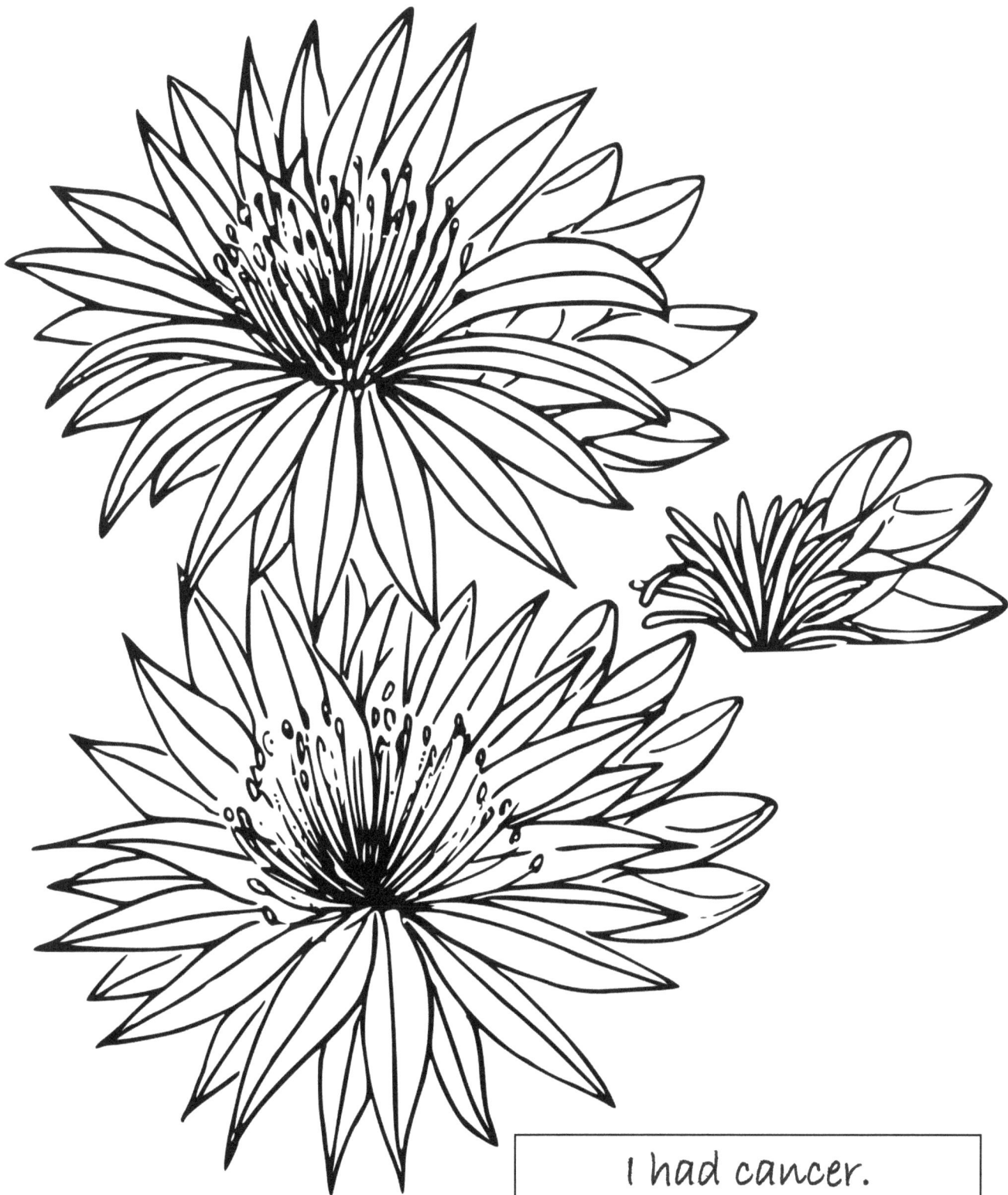

I had cancer.

Cancer _never_ had me.

Life isn't about waiting for the storm to pass,

it's about learning how to dance in the rain.

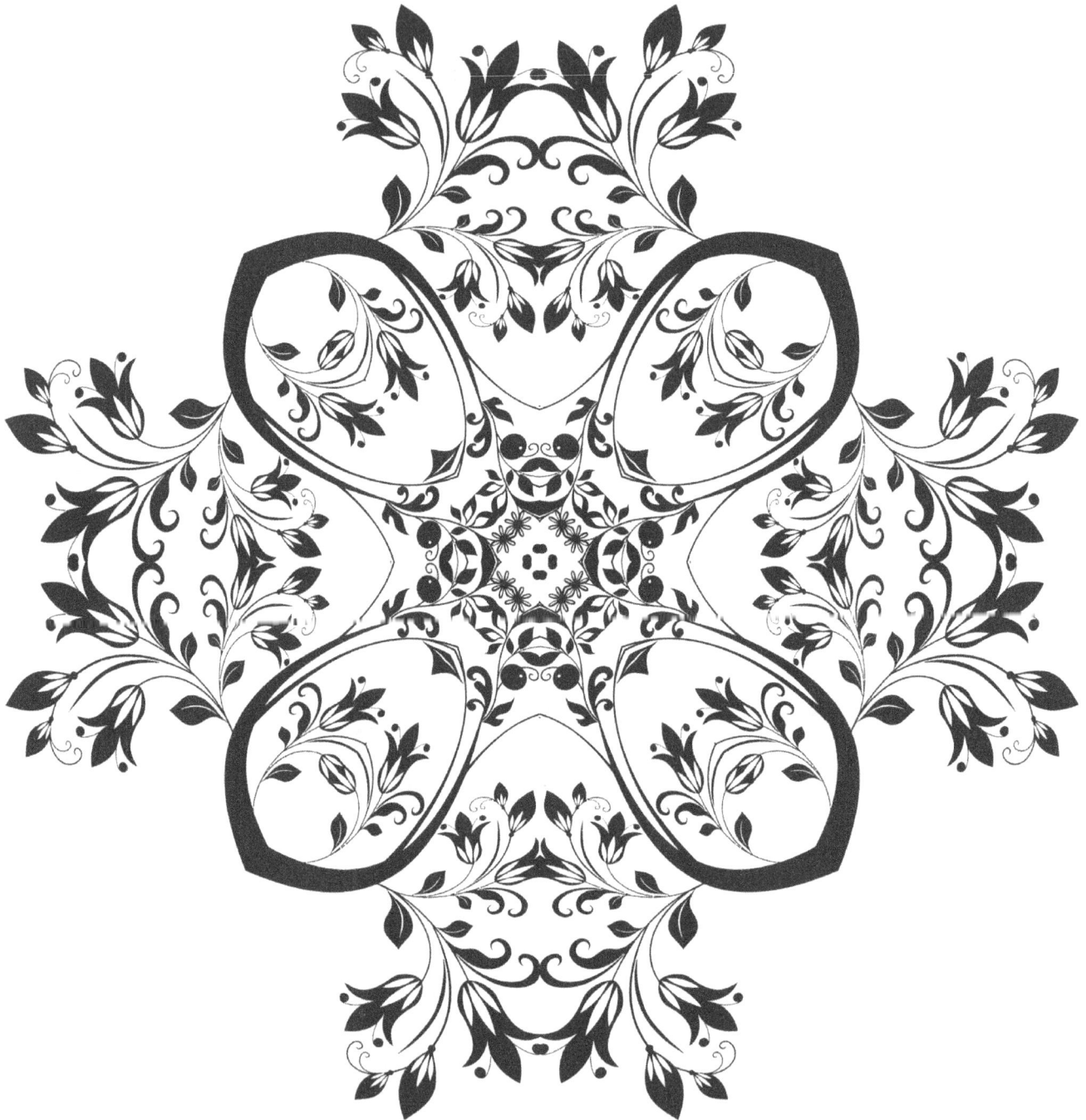

- Lindsay Hodgson

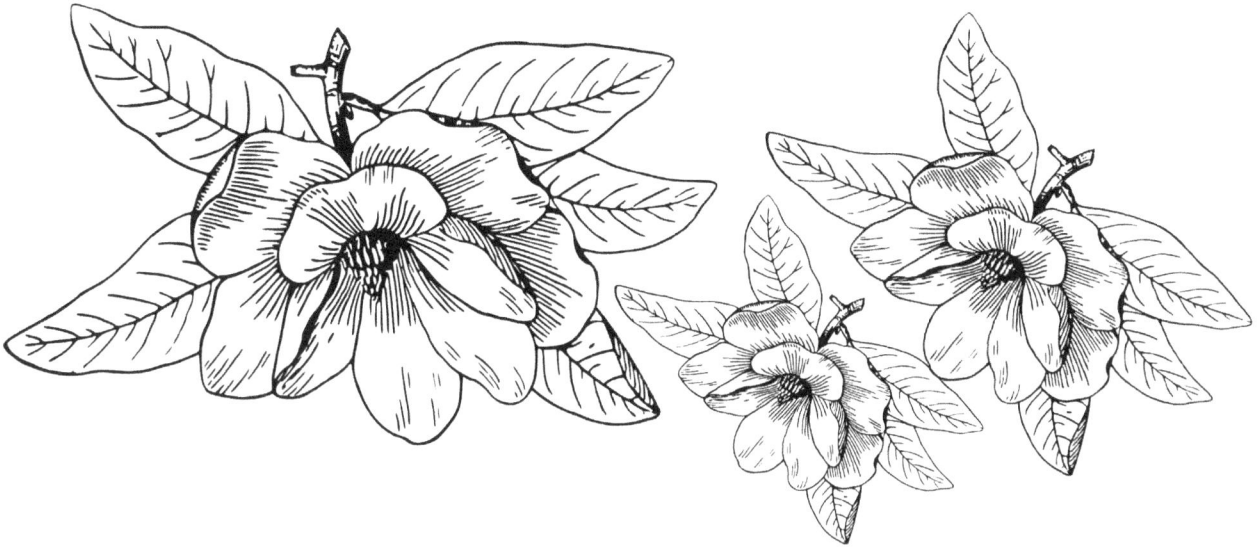

*Courage is not the absence
of fear, but rather the judgment
that something else is more
important than fear.*
- Ambrose Redmoon

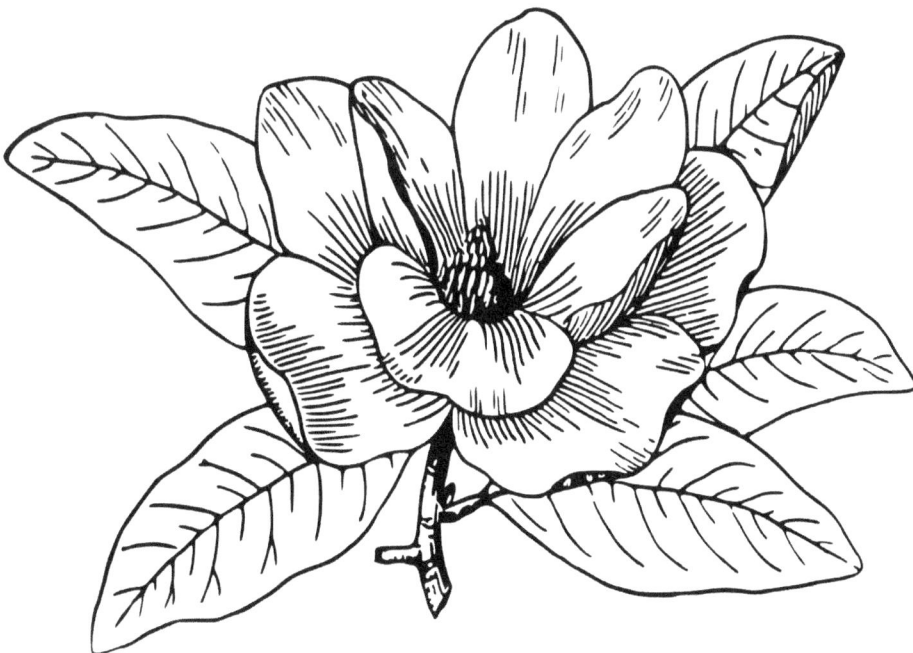

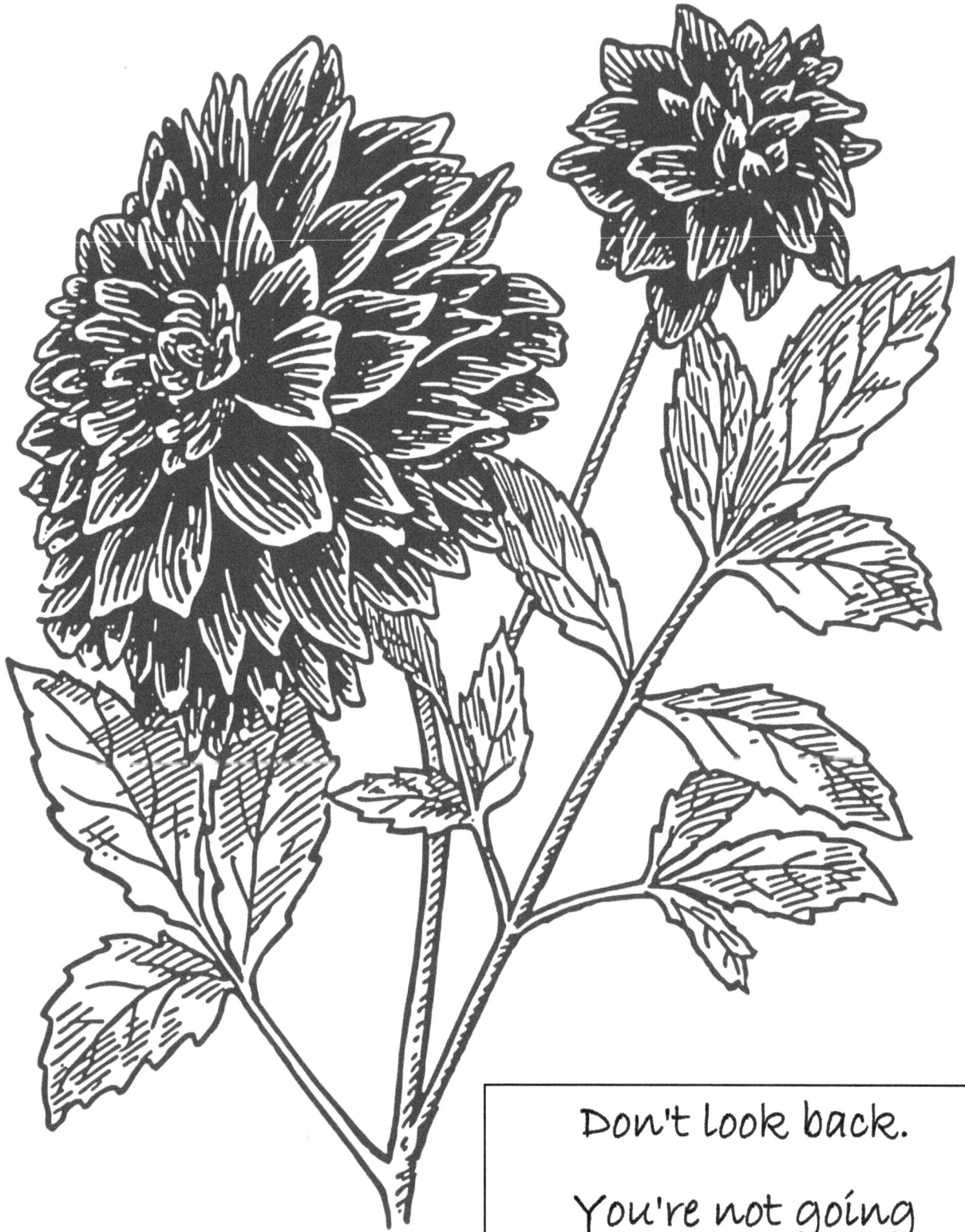

Don't look back.
You're not going
that way.

We cannot direct the wind . . .

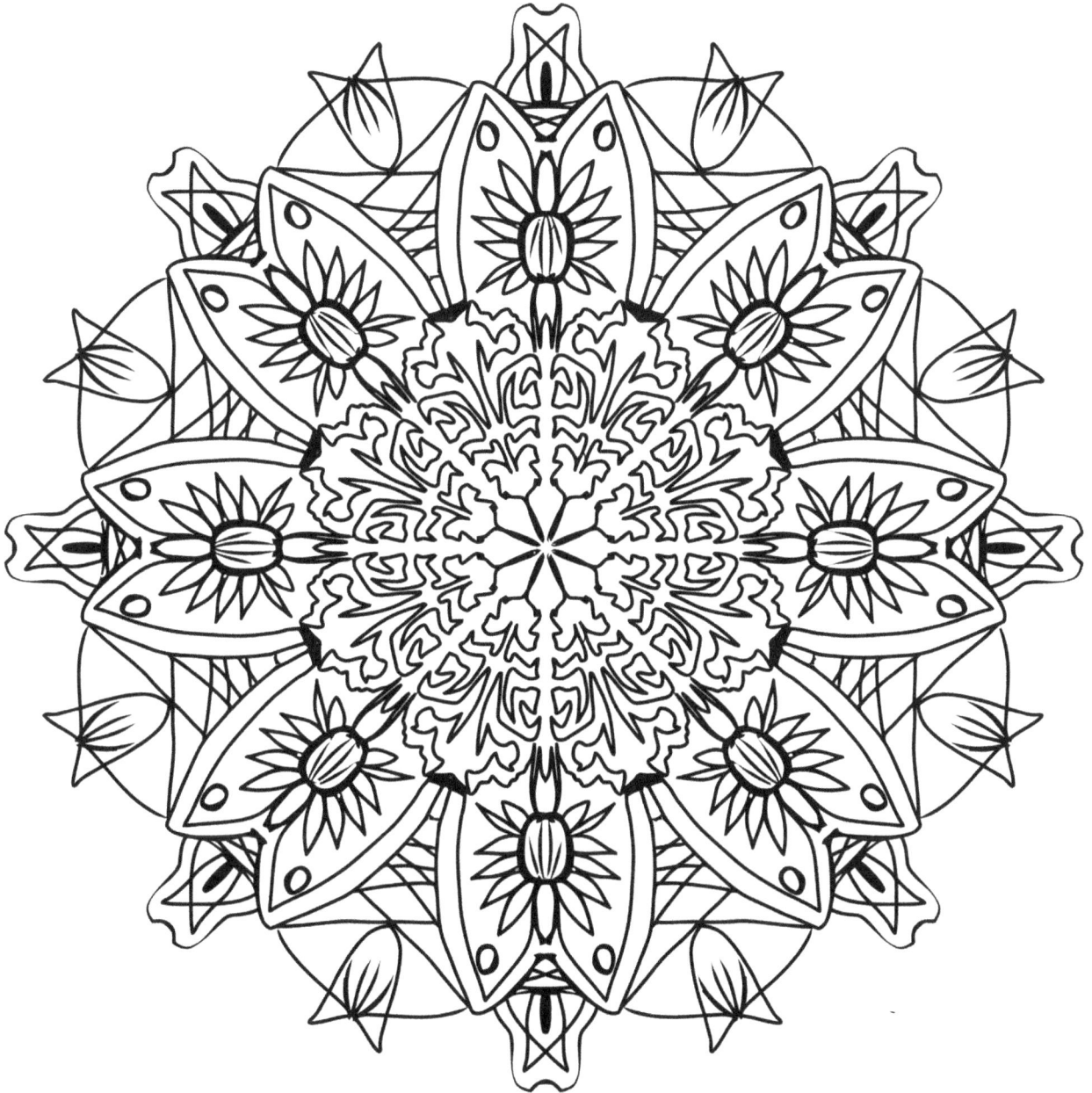

. . . but we can adjust the sails.

Good . thoughts .
only.

Hope is grief's
best music.

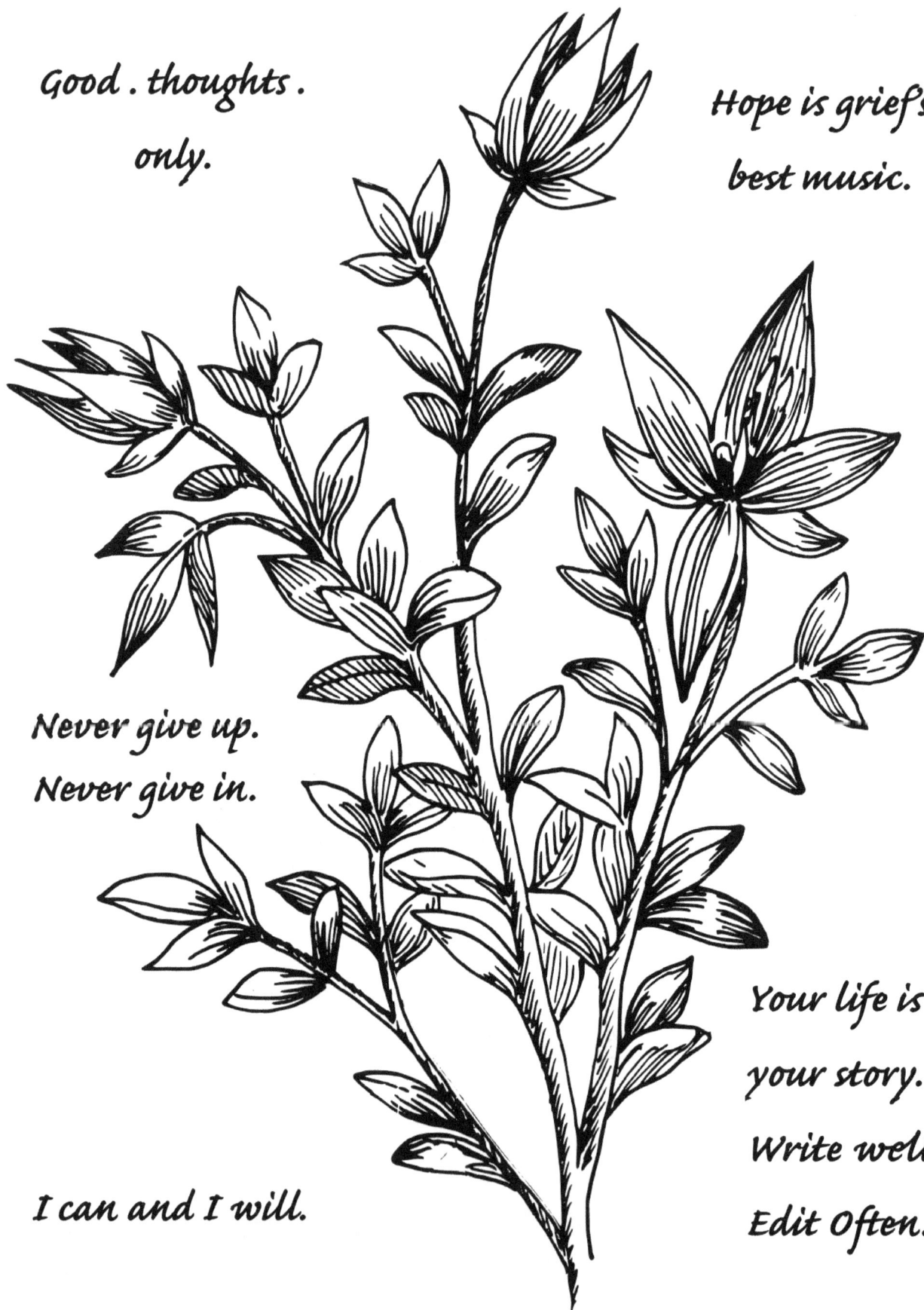

Never give up.
Never give in.

Your life is
your story.
Write well.
Edit Often.

I can and I will.

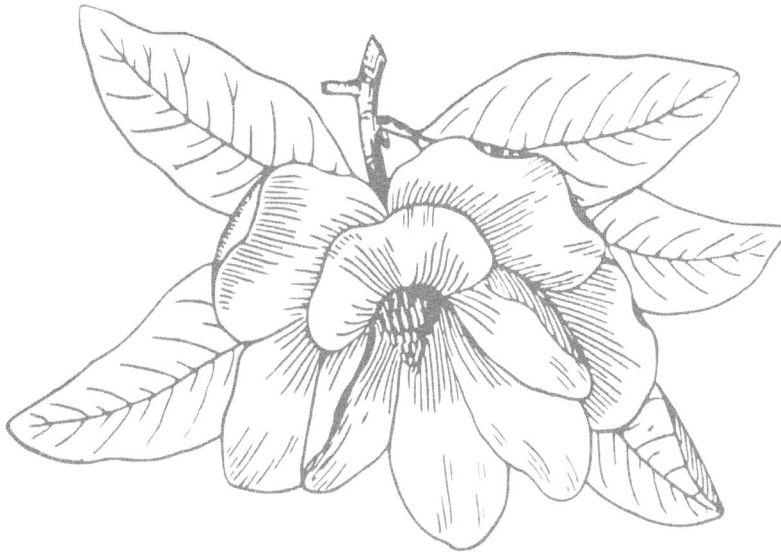

When you have exhausted all possibilities, remember this:

You haven't.

– Thomas Edison

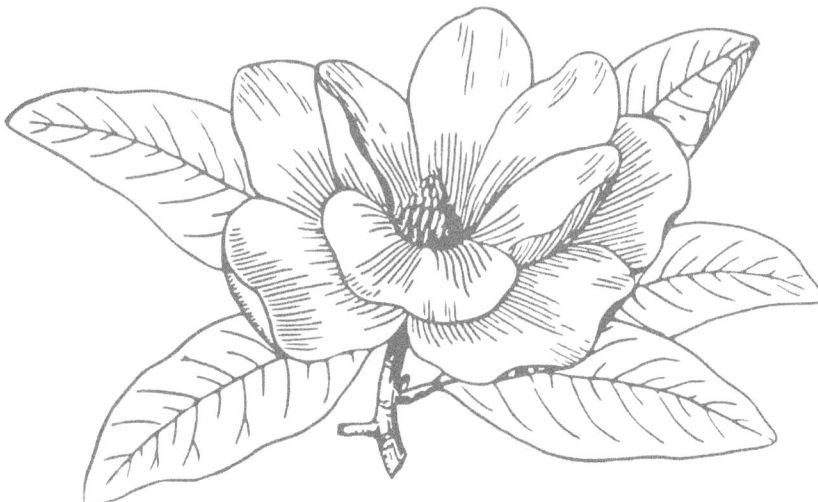

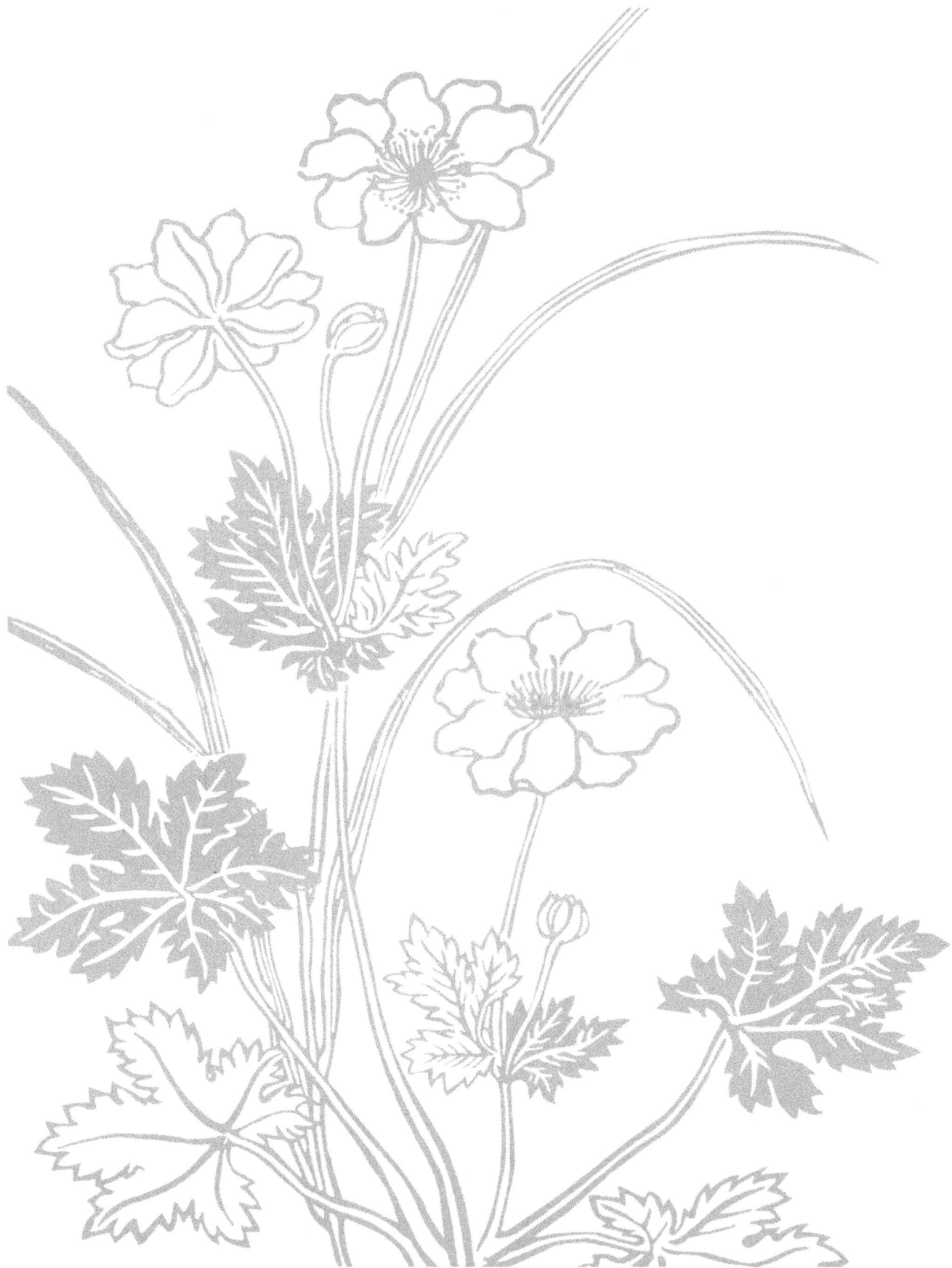

Other books available by the author on Amazon

Journals

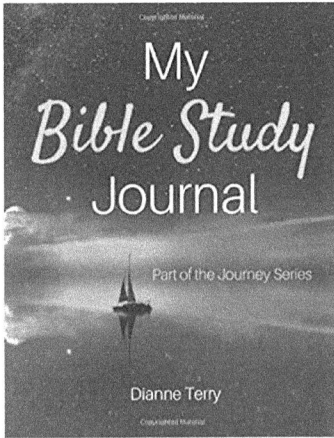

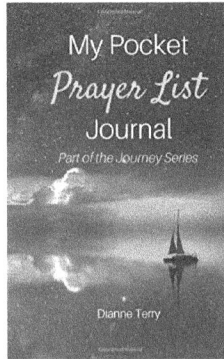

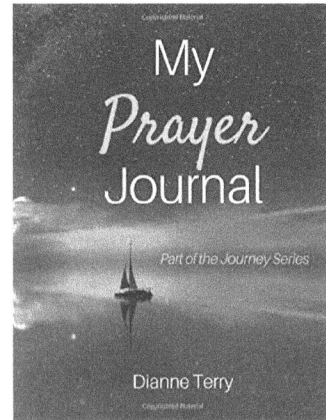

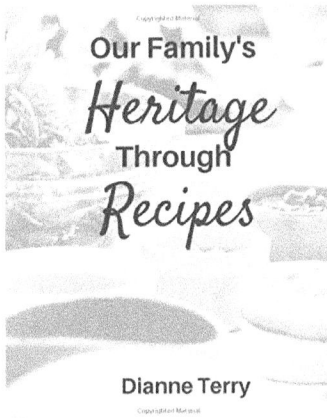

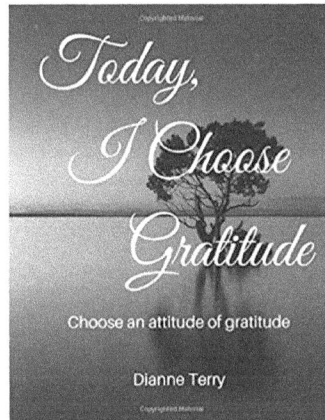

www.ingramcontent.com/pod-product-compliance
Lightning Source LLC
Chambersburg PA
CBHW061617210326
41520CB00041B/7478